HESI A2 Exam Prep and Practice Test Questions Book for the HESI A2 Exam

280+ Exam Practice Questions & Dumps with Explanations

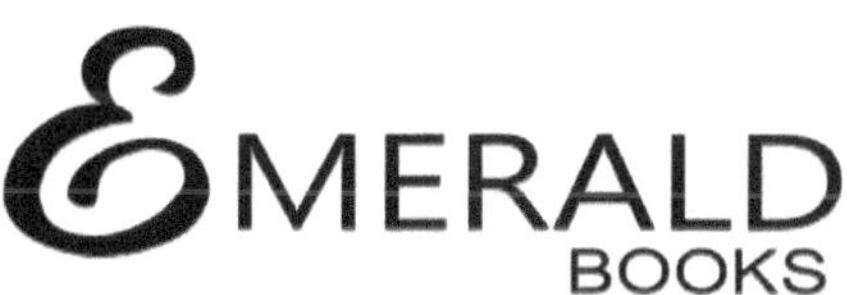

Presented By: Emerald Books

Copyright © 2020 by Emerald Books

First Copy Printed in 2020

About Emerald Books:

Emerald Books is a publishing house based in Hudson, Texas, USA, a platform that is available both online & locally, which unleashes the power of educational content, literary collection, poetry & many other book genres. We make it easy for writers & authors to get their books designed, published, promoted, and sell professionally on worldwide scale with eBook + Print distribution. Emerald Books was founded in 2015, and is now distributing books worldwide.

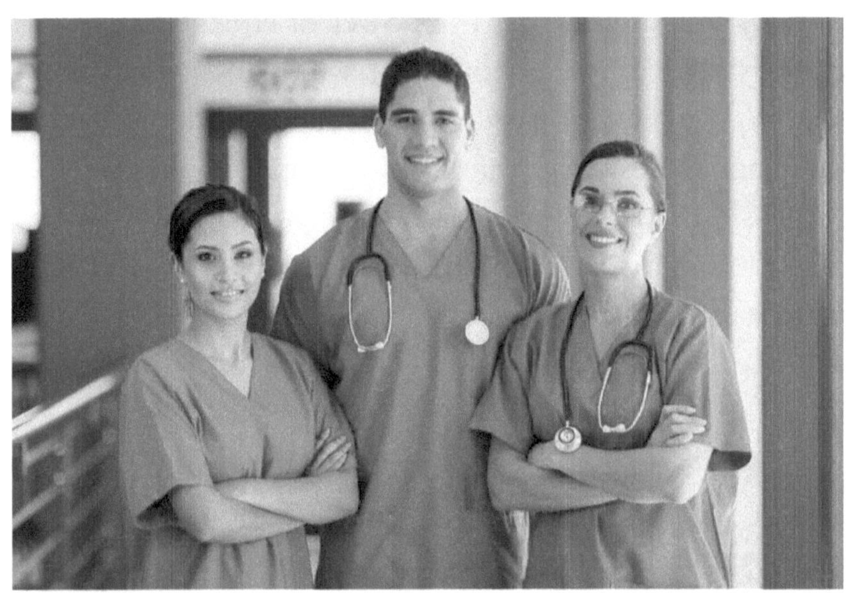

QUESTION 1

A middle-aged woman tells the nurse that she has been experiencing irregular menses for the past six months. The nurse should assess the woman for other symptoms of:

A. climacteric.
B. menopause.
C. perimenopause.
D. postmenopause.

Correct Answer: C

Explanation/Reference:

Perimenopause refers to a period of time in which hormonal changes occur gradually, ovarian function diminishes, and menses become irregular. Perimenopause lasts approximately five years. Climacteric is a term applied to the period of life in which physiologic changes occur and result in cessation of a woman's reproductive ability and lessened sexual activity in males. The term applies to both genders. Climacteric and menopause are interchangeable terms when used for females. Menopause is the period when permanent cessation of menses has occurred. Postmenopause refers to the period after the changes accompanying menopause are complete. Health Promotion and Maintenance

QUESTION 2

When obtaining a health history on a menopausal woman, which information should a nurse recognize as a contraindication for hormone replacement therapy?

A. family history of stroke
B. ovaries removed before age 45
C. frequent hot flashes and/or night sweats
D. unexplained vaginal bleeding

Correct Answer: D

Explanation/Reference:

Unexplained vaginal bleeding is a contraindication for hormone replacement therapy. Family history of stroke is not a contraindication for hormone replacement therapy. If the woman herself had a history of stroke or
other blood-clotting events, hormone therapy could be contraindicated. Frequent hot flashes and/or night sweats can be relieved by hormone replacement therapy. Health Promotion and Maintenance

QUESTION 3

Teaching about the need to avoid foods high in potassium is most important for which client?

A. a client receiving diuretic therapy
B. a client with an ileostomy

C. a client with metabolic alkalosis

D. a client with renal disease

Correct Answer: D

Explanation/Reference:

Clients with renal disease are predisposed to hyperkalemia and should
avoid foods high in potassium. Choices 1, 2, and 3 are incorrect
because clients receiving diuretics with ileostomy or with metabolic
alkalosis are at risk for hypokalemia and should be encouraged to eat
foods high in potassium. Physiological Adaptation

QUESTION 4

What do the following ABG values indicate: pH 7.38, PO2 78 mmHg,
PCO2 36mmHg, and HCO3 24 mEq/ L?

A. metabolic alkalosis

B. homeostasis

C. respiratory acidosis

D. respiratory alkalosis

Correct Answer: B

Explanation/Reference:

These ABG values are within normal limits. Choices 1, 3, and 4 are
incorrect because the ABG values indicate none of these acid-base
disturbances. Physiological Adaptation

QUESTION 5

The major electrolytes in the extracellular fluid are:

A. potassium and chloride.

B. potassium and phosphate.

C. sodium and chloride.

D. sodium and phosphate.

Correct Answer: C

Explanation/Reference:

Sodium and chloride are the major electrolytes in the extracellular fluid.
Physiological Adaptation

QUESTION 6

A client with Kawasaki disease has bilateral congestion of the
conjunctivae, dry cracked lips, a strawberry tongue, and edema of the
hands and feet followed by desquamation of fingers and toes. Which of
the following nursing measures is most appropriate to meet the
expected outcome of positive body image?

A. administering immune globulin intravenously
B. assessing the extremities for edema, redness and desquamation
   every 8 hours

C. explaining progression of the disease to the client and his or her
   family
D. assessing heart sounds and rhythm

Correct Answer: C

Explanation/Reference:

Teaching the client and family about progression of the disease
includes explaining when symptoms can be expected to improve and
resolve. Knowledge of the course of the disease can help them
understand that no
permanent disruption in physical appearance will occur that could
negatively affect body image. Clients with
Kawasaki disease might receive immune globulin intravenously to
reduce the incidence of coronary artery lesions
and aneurysms. Cardiac effects could be linked to body image, but
Choice 3 is the most direct link to body image.
The nurse assesses symptoms to assist in evaluation of treatment and
progression of the disease.Health Promotion and Maintenance

QUESTION 7

Which of the following is most likely to impact the body image of an
infant newly diagnosed with Hemophilia?

A. immobility
B. altered growth and development

C. hemarthrosis

D. altered family processes

Correct Answer: D

Explanation/Reference:

Altered Family Processes is a potential nursing diagnosis for the family
and client with a new diagnosis of Hemophilia. Infants are aware of
how their caregivers respond to their needs. Stresses can have an
immediate impact on the infant's development of trust and how others
relate to them because of their diagnosis.

The long term effects of hemophilia can include problems related to
immobility. Altered growth and development could not have developed
in a newly diagnosed client. Hemarthrosis is acute bleeding into a joint
space that is characteristic of hemophilia. It does not have an
immediate effect on the body image of a newly diagnosed hemophiliac.
Health Promotion and Maintenance

QUESTION 8

While undergoing fetal heart monitoring, a pregnant Native-American
woman requests that a medicine woman be present in the examination
room. Which of the following is an appropriate response by the nurse?

A. "I will assist you in arranging to have a medicine woman present."
B. "We do not allow medicine women in exam rooms."
C. "That does not make any difference in the outcome."
D. "It is old-fashioned to believe in that."

Correct Answer: A

Explanation/Reference:

This statement reflects cultural awareness and acceptance that
receiving support from a medicine woman is important to the client.
The other statements are culturally insensitive and unprofessional.
Reduction of Risk Potential

QUESTION 9

All of the following should be performed when fetal heart monitoring
indicates fetal distress except:

A. increase maternal fluids.
B. administer oxygen.
C. decrease maternal fluids.
D. turn the mother.

Correct Answer: C

Explanation/Reference:

Decreasing maternal fluids is the only intervention that should not be
performed when fetal distress is indicated. Reduction of Risk Potential

QUESTION 10

Which fetal heart monitor pattern can indicate cord compression?

A. variable decelerations
B. early decelerations
C. bradycardia
D. tachycardia

Correct Answer: A

Explanation/Reference:

Variable decelerations can be related to cord compression. The other
patterns are not.Reduction of Risk Potential

QUESTION 11

Which of the following conditions is mammography used to detect?

A. pain
B. tumor
C. edema
D. epilepsy

Correct Answer: B

Explanation/Reference:

Mammography is used to detect tumors or cysts in the breasts, not the other conditions. Reduction of Risk Potential

QUESTION 12

Why might breast implants interfere with mammography?

A. They might cause additional discomfort.
B. They are contraindications to mammography.
C. They are likely to be dislodged.
D. They might prevent detection of masses.

Correct Answer: D

Explanation/Reference:

Breast implants can prevent detection of masses. Choices 1, 2, and 3 are not ways in which breast implants interfere with mammography. Reduction of Risk Potential

QUESTION 13

Which of the following instructions should the nurse give a client who will be undergoing mammography?

A. Be sure to use underarm deodorant.
B. Do not use underarm deodorant.
C. Do not eat or drink after midnight.
D. Have a friend drive you home.

Correct Answer: B

Explanation/Reference:

Underarm deodorant should not be used because it might cause confusing shadows on the X-ray film.
There are no restrictions on food or fluid intake. No sedation is used, so the client can drive herself home. Reduction of Risk Potential

QUESTION 14

Which of the following diseases or conditions is least likely to be associated with increased potential for bleeding?

A. metastatic liver cancer
B. gram-negative septicemia
C. pernicious anemia
D. iron-deficiency anemia

Correct Answer: C

Explanation/Reference:

Pernicious anemia results from vitamin B12 deficiency due to lack of intrinsic factor. This can result from inadequate dietary intake, faulty absorption from the GI tract due to a lack of secretion of intrinsic factor normally produced by gastric mucosal cells and certain disorders of the small intestine that impair absorption.

The nurse should instruct the client in the need for lifelong replacement of vitamin B12, as well as the need for folic acid, rest, diet, and support. Physiological Adaptation

QUESTION 15

A client has been diagnosed with Disseminated Intravascular Coagulation (DIC) and transferred to the medical intensive care unit (ICU) subsequent to an acute bleeding episode. In the ICU, continuous Heparin drip therapy is initiated. Which of the following assessment findings indicates a positive response to Heparin therapy?

A. increased platelet count
B. increased fibrinogen
C. decreased fibrin split products
D. decreased bleeding

Correct Answer: B

Explanation/Reference:

Effective Heparin therapy should stop the process of intravascular coagulation and result in increased availability of fibrinogen. Heparin administration interferes with thrombin-induced conversion of fibrinogen to fibrin. Bleeding should cease due to the increased availability of platelets and coagulation factors. Physiological Adaptation

QUESTION 16

A client, age 28, was recently diagnosed with Hodgkin's disease. After staging, therapy is planned to include combination radiation therapy and systemic chemotherapy with MOPP-- nitrogen mustard, vincristine (Onconvin), prednisone, and procarbazine. In planning care for this client, the nurse should anticipate which of the following side effects to contribute to a sense of altered body image?

A. cushingoid appearance
B. alopecia
C. temporary or permanent sterility
D. pathologic fractures

Correct Answer: D

Explanation/Reference:

Pathologic fractures are not common to the disease process. Its treatment through osteoporosis is a potential complication of steroid use. Hodgkin's disease most commonly affects young adults (males), is spread through lymphatic channels to contiguous nodes, and also might spread via the hematogenous route to extradal sites (GI, bone marrow, skin, and other organs). A working staging classification is performed for clinical use and care. Physiological Adaptation

QUESTION 17

Which of the following is an inappropriate item to include in planning care for a severely neutropenic client?

A. Transfuse netrophils (granulocytes) to prevent infection.
B. Exclude raw vegetables from the diet.
C. Avoid administering rectal suppositories.
D. Prohibit vases of fresh flowers and plants in the client's room.

Correct Answer: A

Explanation/Reference:

Granulocyte transfusion is not indicated to prevent infection. Produced in the bone marrow, granulocytes normally comprise 70% of all WBCs. They are subdivided into three types based on staining properties: neutrophils, eosinophils, and basophils. They can be beneficial in a selected population of infected, severely granulocytopenic clients (less than 500/mm3) who do not respond to antibiotic therapy and who are expected to experience prolonged suppression of granulocyte production. Physiological Adaptation

QUESTION 18

Which sign might the nurse see in a client with a high ammonia level?

A. coma
B. edema
C. hypoxia
D. polyuria

Correct Answer: A

Explanation/Reference:

Coma might be seen in a client with a high ammonia level. Reduction of Risk Potential

QUESTION 19

A Client with which of the following conditions is at risk for developing a high ammonia level?

A. renal failure
B. psoriasis
C. lupus
D. cirrhosis

Correct Answer: D

Explanation/Reference:

A client with cirrhosis is at risk for developing a high ammonia level. Reduction of Risk Potential

QUESTION 20

For which of the following conditions might blood be drawn for uric acid level?

A. asthma
B. gout
C. diverticulitis
D. meningitis

Correct Answer: B

Explanation/Reference:

Uric acid levels are indicated for clients with gout. Reduction of Risk Potential

QUESTION 21

Which of the following foods might a client with a hypercholesterolemia need to decrease his or her intake of?

A. broiled catfish
B. hamburgers
C. wheat bread
D. fresh apples

Correct Answer: B

Explanation/Reference:

Due to the high cholesterol content of red meats, such as hamburger, intake needs to be decreased. The other options do not have high cholesterol content, so they do not need to be decreased. Reduction of Risk Potential

QUESTION 22

Which of the following lab values is associated with a decreased risk of cardiovascular disease?

A. high HDL cholesterol
B. low HDL cholesterol
C. low total cholesterol
D. low triglycerides

Correct Answer: A

Explanation/Reference:

High HDL cholesterol and low LDL cholesterol are associated with a decreased risk of cardiovascular disease. Reduction of Risk Potential

QUESTION 23

Which of the following organs of the digestive system has a primary function of absorption?

A. stomach
B. pancreas

C. small intestine
D. gallbladder

Correct Answer: C

Explanation/Reference:

The small intestine has a primary function of absorption. The remaining digestive organs have other primary functions. Physiological Adaptation

QUESTION 24

For a client with suspected appendicitis, the nurse should expect to find abdominal tenderness in which quadrant?

A. upper right
B. upper left
C. lower right
D. lower left

Correct Answer: C

Explanation/Reference:

The nurse should expect to find abdominal tenderness in the lower-right quadrant in a client with appendicitis.
Physiological Adaptation

QUESTION 25

A 20-year-old obese female client is preparing to have gastric bypass surgery for weight loss. She says to the nurse, "I need this surgery because nothing else I have done has helped me to lose weight." Which response by the nurse is most appropriate?

A. "If you eat less, you can save some money."
B. "Exercise is a healthier way to lose weight."
C. "You should try the Atkins diet first."
D. "I respect your decision to choose surgery."

Correct Answer: D

Explanation/Reference:

This statement is most appropriate, as it shows respect and empathy.
The other statements are both insensitive and unprofessional.
Physiological Adaptation

QUESTION 26

A client with an ileus is placed on intestinal tube suction. Which of the
following electrolytes is lost with intestinal suction?

A. calcium
B. magnesium
C. potassium
D. sodium chloride

Correct Answer: D

Explanation/Reference:

Duodenal intestinal fluid is rich in K+, NA+, and bicarbonate.
Suctioning to remove excess fluids decreases the client's K+ and NA+
levels. Basic Care and Comfort

QUESTION 27

Following a classic cholecystectomy resection for multiple stones, the
PACU nurse observes a serosanguious drainage on the dressing. The
most appropriate intervention is to:

A. notify the physician of the drainage.
B. change the dressing.
C. reinforce the dressing.
D. apply an abdominal binder.

Correct Answer: C

Explanation/Reference:

Serosanguious drainage is expected at this time. The dressing should be reinforced. Changing a new postop dressing increases the risk of infection. An abdominal binder interferes with visualization of the dressing. Basic Care and Comfort

QUESTION 28

A client who is immobilized secondary to traction is complaining of constipation. Which of the following medications should the nurse expect to be ordered?

A. Advil
B. Anasaid
C. Clinocil
D. Colace

Correct Answer: D

Explanation/Reference:

Colace is a stool softener that acts by pulling more water into the bowel lumen, making the stool soft and easier to evacuate. Basic Care and Comfort

QUESTION 29

A client is complaining of difficulty walking secondary to a mass in the foot. The nurse should document this finding as:

A. plantar fasciitis.
B. hallux valgus.
C. hammertoe.
D. Morton's neuroma.

Correct Answer: D

Morton's neuroma is a small mass or tumor in a digital nerve of the foot. Hallux valgus is referred to in lay terms as abunion. Hammertoe is where one toe is cocked up over another toe. Plantar fasciitis is an inflammation of, or pain in, the arch of the foot. Basic Care and Comfort

QUESTION 30

A client turns her ankle. She is diagnosed as having a Pulled Ligament. This should be documented as a:

A. sprain.
B. strain.
C. subluxation.
D. distoration.

Correct Answer: B

Explanation/Reference:

A strain is excessive stretching of a ligament. A sprain involves a twisting motion involving muscles.Basic Care and Comfort

QUESTION 31

To remove hard contact lenses from an unresponsive client, the nurse should:

A. gently irrigate the eye with an irrigating solution from the inner canthus outward.
B. grasp the lens with a gentle pinching motion.

C. don sterile gloves before attempting the procedure.
D. ensure that the lens is centered on the cornea before gently
manipulating the lids to release the lens.

Correct Answer: D

Explanation/Reference:

To remove hard contact lenses, the upper and lower eyelids are gently
maneuvered to help loosen the lens and slide it out of the eye. The
lens must be situated on the cornea, not the sclera, before removal. An
attempt to grasp a hard lens might result in a scratch on the cornea.
Clean gloves are an option if drainage is present. Basic Care and
Comfort

QUESTION 32

To remove a client's gown when she has an intravenous line, the nurse
should:

A. temporarily disconnect the intravenous tubing at a point close to the
client and thread it through the gown.
B. cut the gown with scissors.
C. thread the bag and tubing through the gown sleeve, keeping the
line intact.
D. temporarily disconnect the tubing from the intravenous container
and thread it through the gown.

Correct Answer: C

Explanation/Reference:

Threading the bag and tubing through the gown sleeve keeps the
system intact. Opening an intravenous line causes a break in a sterile
system and introduces the potential for infection. Cutting a gown off is
not an alternative except in an emergency. IV gowns, which open
along sleeves, are widely available. Basic Care and Comfort

QUESTION 33

When making an occupied bed, it is important for the nurse to:

A. keep the bed in the low position.
B. use a bath blanket or top sheet for warmth and privacy.
C. constantly keep side rails raised on both sides.
D. move back and forth from one side to the other when adjusting the linens.

Correct Answer: B

Explanation/Reference:

Using a bath blanket or top sheet keeps the client warm and provides privacy. Keeping the bed in the low position and working above raised side rails might strain the nurse's back. Continually moving back and forth to tuck and arrange linen is time-consuming and disorganized. Basic Care and Comfort

QUESTION 34

Diagnostic genetic counseling, for procedures such as amniocentesis and chorionic villus sampling, allows clients to make all of the following choices except:

A. terminating the pregnancy.
B. preparing for the birth of a child with special needs.
C. accessing support services before the birth.
D. completing the grieving process before the birth.

Correct Answer: D

Explanation/Reference:

If findings are ominous, the grieving process will not be completed before birth. If the couple elects to terminate a pregnancy based on diagnostic tests, there will be grief and concerns for future pregnancies.

Couples might choose to access support services and prepare for the birth of an infant with special needs. Some fetal conditions can be treated in utero. Health Promotion and Maintenance

QUESTION 35

A client who is experiencing infertility says to the nurse, "I feel I will be incomplete as a man/woman if I cannot have a child." Which of the following nursing diagnoses is likely to be appropriate for this client?

A. Risk for Self Harm
B. Body Image Disturbance
C. Ineffective Role Performance
D. Powerlessness

Correct Answer: B

Explanation/Reference:

Of the nursing diagnoses listed, the client's statement most represents Body Image Disturbance because it directly refers to loss of the function of having a child. Nothing in the statement indicates that the client is at risk for harming herself. Ineffective Role Performance could be correct but is not the best choice because the statement does not reflect a disruption of the parent's role. Powerlessness could be an appropriate nursing diagnosis if the client described feeling powerless about the infertility. Health Promotion and Maintenance

QUESTION 36

Which of the following foods is a complete protein?

A. corn
B. eggs
C. peanutsDsunflower seeds

Correct Answer: B

Explanation/Reference:

Eggs are a complete protein. The remaining options are incomplete proteins. Health Promotion and Maintenance

QUESTION 37

Which condition is associated with inadequate intake of vitamin C?

A. rickets
B. marasmus
C. kwashiorkor
D. scurvy

Correct Answer: D

Explanation/Reference:

Scurvy is associated with inadequate intake of vitamin C. The remaining choices refer to other nutritional deficiencies. Health Promotion and Maintenance

QUESTION 38

What is the primary nutritional deficiency of concern for a strict vegetarian?

A. vitamin C
B. vitamin B12
C. vitamin E
D. magnesium
E.

Correct Answer: B

Explanation/Reference:

Vitamin B12 is the primary nutritional deficiency of concern for a strict vegetarian. Health Promotion and Maintenance

QUESTION 39

How often should the nurse change the intravenous tubing on total parenteral nutrition solutions?

A. every 24 hours
B. every 36 hours
C. every 48 hours
D. every 72 hours

Correct Answer: A

Explanation/Reference:

The nurse should change the intravenous tubing on total parenteral
nutrition solutions every 24 hours, due to the high risk of bacterial
growth. Health Promotion and Maintenance

QUESTION 40

Which of the following values should the nurse monitor closely while a
client is on total parenteral nutrition?

A. calcium
B. magnesium
C. glucose
D. cholesterol

Correct Answer: C

Explanation/Reference:

Glucose is monitored closely when a client is on total parenteral
nutrition, due to high glucose concentration in the solutions. The other
values are not monitored as closely. Health Promotion and
Maintenance

QUESTION 41

A teenage client is admitted to the hospital because of acetaminophen
(Tylenol) overdose. Overdoses of acetaminophen can precipitate life-
threatening abnormalities in which of the following organs?

A. lungs

B. liver
C. kidneys
D. adrenal glands

Correct Answer: B

Explanation/Reference:

Acetaminophen is extensively metabolized in the liver. Choices 1, 3, and 4 are incorrect because prolonged use of acetaminophen might result in an increased risk of renal dysfunction, but a single overdose does not precipitate life-threatening problems in the respiratory system, renal system, or adrenal glands. Pharmacological Therapies

QUESTION 42

Light therapy can be effective for:

A. overcoming weight problems.
B. helping with allergies.
C. use in alternative medical treatments.
D. working with sleep patterns.

Correct Answer: D

Explanation/Reference:

Light therapy can be effective in treating problems associated with sleep patterns, stress, moods, jaundice in newborns, and seasonal affective disorders. Non pharmacological Therapies

QUESTION 43

Broccoli, oranges, dark greens, and dark yellow vegetables can be eaten to:

A. supplement vitamin pills.
B. balance body molecules.
C. cure many diseases.
D. help improve body defenses.

Correct Answer: D

Explanation/Reference:

Controversy over what types of food to eat and not eat is still under investigation. Certain foods can help improve body defenses to possibly prevent certain diseases. Non pharmacological Therapies

QUESTION 44

A diet high in fiber content can help an individual to:

A. lose body weight fast.
B. reduce diabetic ketoacidosis.
C. lower cholesterol.
D. reduce the need for folate.

Correct Answer: C

Explanation/Reference:

Fiber-rich foods (such as grains, apples, potatoes, and beans) can help lower cholesterol. Non pharmacological Therapies

QUESTION 45

Which of the following is an appropriate nursing goal for a client at risk for nutritional problems?

A. provide oxygen
B. promote healthy nutritional practices
C. treat complications of malnutrition
D. increase weight

Correct Answer: B

Explanation/Reference:

Promoting healthy nutritional practices is an appropriate nursing goal for a client at risk for nutritional problems. Choice 1 is incorrect because it is a nursing intervention, not a goal statement. Choice 3 is incorrect because it is a therapeutic treatment. Choice 4 is incorrect because weight gain is an appropriate goal only if the client is underweight. Basic Care and Comfort

QUESTION 46

The nurse explains to a client who underwent gastric resection that which of the following meals is most likely to cause rapid emptying of the stomach?

A. a high-protein meal
B. a high-fat meal
C. a large meal regardless of nutrient content
D. a high-carbohydrate meal

Correct Answer: D

Explanation/Reference:

Meals that are high in carbohydrates promote rapid gastric emptying. The other options are associated with decreased emptying time. Basic Care and Comfort

QUESTION 47

Which of the following foods should be avoided by clients who are prone to develop heartburn as a result of gastroesophgeal reflux disease (GERD)?

A. lettuce
B. eggs
C. chocolate
D. butterscotch

Correct Answer: C

Explanation/Reference:

Ingestion of chocolate can reduce lower esophageal sphincter (LES) pressure leading to reflux and clinical symptoms of GERD. The other foods do not affect LES pressure. Basic Care and Comfort

QUESTION 48

Nurses caring for clients who have cancer and are taking opioids need to assess for all of the following except:

A. tolerance.
B. constipation.
C. sedation.
D. addiction.

Correct Answer: D

Explanation/Reference:

Addiction is not of primary concern when treating the pain of terminally ill clients. Clients with cancer who are taking opioid analgesics can develop tolerance, constipation, and sedation. Basic Care and Comfort

QUESTION 49

The goals of palliative care include all of the following except:

A. giving clients with life-threatening illnesses the best quality of life possible.
B. taking care of the whole person--body, mind, spirit, heart, and soul.
C. no interventions are needed because the client is near death.
D. support of needs of the family and client.

Correct Answer: C

Explanation/Reference:

The goals of palliative care include choices 1, 2, and 4. Choice 3 is not part of palliative care. All aspects of medical, emotional, social, and spiritual needs of the dying client should be focused on until the end of life.Basic Care and Comfort

QUESTION 50

Major competencies for the nurse giving end-of life care include:

A. demonstrating respect and compassion, and applying knowledge and skills in care of the family and the client.
B. assessing and intervening to support total management of the family and client.

C. setting goals, expectations, and dynamic changes to care for the client.
D. keeping all sad news away from the family and client.

Correct Answer: A

Explanation/Reference:

There are many competencies that the nurse must have to care for families and clients at the end of life. Demonstration of respect and compassion as well as using knowledge and skills in the care of the client and family are major competencies. Basic Care and Comfort

QUESTION 51

Assessment of the client with an arteriovenous fistula for hemodialysis should include:

A. inspection for visible pulsation.
B. palpation of thrill.
C. percussion for dullness.
D. auscultation of blood pressure.

Correct Answer: B

Explanation/Reference:

Thrill should be present. The client should be taught to check this daily at home. Pulsation is not typically visible. Percussion gives no information about the patency of a fistula. Blood pressure is not auscultated in a limb with an AVF. Auscultation of the AVF, for a bruit, is part of an assessment for patency. Physiological Adaptation

QUESTION 52

A client has been taking alprazolam (Xanax) for four years to manage anxiety. The client reports taking 0.5 mg four times a day. Which statement indicates that the client understands the nurse's teaching about discontinuing the medication?

A. "I can drink alcohol now that I am decreasing my Xanax."
B. "I should not take another Xanax pill. Here is what is left of my last prescription."

C. "I should take three pills per day next week, then two pills for one week, then one pill for one week."
D. "I can expect to be sleepy for several days after stopping the medicine."

Correct Answer: C

Explanation/Reference:

Xanax, like other benzodiazepines, can cause withdrawal symptoms that include agitation, insomnia, hypertension, seizures, and abdominal pain. The drug must be slowly decreased to prevent withdrawal symptoms. Psychosocial Integrity

QUESTION 53

A 10-month-old child is brought to the Emergency Department because he is difficult to awaken. The nurse notes bruises on both upper arms. These findings are most consistent with:

A. wearing clothing that is too small for the child.
B. the child being shaken.
C. falling while learning to walk.
D. parents trying to awaken the child.

Correct Answer: B

Explanation/Reference:

Children who are shaken are frequently grasped by both upper arms. Symptoms of brain injury associated with shaking include decreased level of consciousness. Psychosocial Integrity

QUESTION 54

A health care worker is concerned about a new mother being overwhelmed by caring for her infant. The health care worker should:

A. immediately contact child protective services.
B. provide the mother with literature about child care.
C. consult a therapist to help the mother work out her fears.
D. refer the mother to parenting classes.

Correct Answer: D

Explanation/Reference:

Prevention of child abuse is centered on teaching the parents how to care for their child and cope with the demands of infant care. Parenting classes can help build self-confidence, self-esteem, and coping skills. Parents benefit by understanding the developmental needs of their children, while learning how to manage their home environment more effectively. The classes also increase the parents' social contacts and teach about community resources. Psychosocial Integrity

QUESTION 55

Which of the following methods of contraception is able to reduce the transmission of HIV and other STDs?

A. intrauterine device (IUD)
B. Norplant
C. oral contraceptives
D. vaginal sponge

Correct Answer: D

Explanation/Reference:

The vaginal sponge is a barrier method of contraception that, when used with foam or jelly contraception, reduces the transmission of HIV and other STDs as well as reducing the risk of pregnancy. IUDs, Norplant, and oral contraceptives can prevent pregnancy but not the transmission HIV and STDs. Clients using the contraceptive methods in Choices 1, 2, and 3 should be counseled to use a chemical or barrier contraceptive to decrease transmission of HIV or STDs. Health Promotion and Maintenance

QUESTION 56

Which of the following is the primary force in sex education in a child's life?

A. school nurse
B. peers
C. parents
D. media

Correct Answer: C

Explanation/Reference:

Parents are the primary force in sex education in a child's life. The school nurse is involved with formal sex education and counseling. Peers become more important in sex education during adolescence but might lack correct information. The media play a powerful role in what children learn about sex through movies, TV, and video games. Health Promotion and Maintenance

QUESTION 57

Which of the following nursing actions is most effective when evaluating a kinetic family drawing?

A. telling the child to draw their family doing something
B. offering specific suggestions of what to include in the drawing
C. discouraging the child from talking about the drawing
D. noting the omission of any family members

Correct Answer: D

Explanation/Reference:

There are several guidelines for evaluating kinetic family drawings, including Choice 4. Effective nursing actions include asking the child to explain what each family member is doing, encouraging him or her to tell as much as possible about the drawing, noting physical intimacy or distance, noting placement of family members in the drawing, noting facial expressions of family members and noting if they are facing each other or turned away.
Choice 1 is initial instruction, not evaluation. Only general encouragement should be given to avoid suggesting themes to the child. Health Promotion and Maintenance

QUESTION 58

All of the following factors, when identified in the history of a family, are correlated with poverty except:

A. high infant mortality rate.
B. frequent use of Emergency Departments.
C. consultation with folk healers.
D. low incidence of dental problems.

Correct Answer: D

Explanation/Reference:

Dental problems are prevalent because of the lack of preventive care and access to care. High infant mortality is one of the most significant problems correlated with poverty. Pregnant women who do not have access to care might come to the Emergency Department when in labor. Those in poverty are likely to use Emergency Departments because they may not be turned away. Those in poverty might also turn to folk healers or other persons in their community for care who might be easier to access and might not demand payment. Health Promotion and Maintenance

QUESTION 59

A client is having a seizure; his blood oxygen saturation drops from 92% to 82%. What should the nurse do first?

A. Open the airway.

B. Administer oxygen.
C. Suction the client.
D. Check for breathing.

Correct Answer: A

Explanation/Reference:

The nurse needs to open the airway first when the oxygen saturation drops. The other actions might be appropriate, but the airway must be patent. Reduction of Risk Potential

QUESTION 60

Which of the following might be an appropriate nursing diagnosis for an epileptic client?

A. Dysreflexia
B. Risk for Injury
C. Urinary Retention
D. Unbalanced Nutrition

Correct Answer: B

Explanation/Reference:

The epileptic client is at risk for injury due to the complications of seizure activity, such as possible head trauma associated with a fall. The other choices are not related to the question. Reduction of Risk Potential

QUESTION 61

A young boy is recently diagnosed with a seizure disorder. Which of the following statements by the boy's mother indicates a need for further teaching by the nurse?

A. "I should make sure he gets plenty of rest."

B. "I should get him a medic alert bracelet."
C. "I should lay him on his back during a seizure."
D. "I should loosen his clothing during a seizure."

Correct Answer: C

Explanation/Reference:

A client having a seizure should be turned to the side to prevent aspiration of secretions. The other statements are correct and indicate adequate understanding of teaching. Reduction of Risk Potential

QUESTION 62

Which of the following nursing diagnoses might be appropriate as Parkinson's disease progresses and complications develop?

A. Impaired Physical Mobility
B. Dysreflexia
C. Hypothermia
D. Impaired Dentition

Correct Answer: A

Explanation/Reference:

The client with Parkinson's disease can develop a shuffling gait and rigidity, causing impaired physical mobility. The other diagnoses do not necessarily relate to a client with Parkinson's disease. Reduction of Risk Potential

QUESTION 63

Which of the following neurological disorders is characterized by writhing, twisting movements of the face and limbs?

A. epilepsy
B. Parkinson's
C. muscular sclerosis
D. Huntington's chorea

Correct Answer: D

Explanation/Reference:

Huntington's chorea is characterized by writhing, twisting movements
of the face and limbs. The remaining options are neurological disorders
that do not have such movements as part of their disease process.
Reduction of Risk Potential

QUESTION 64

Ashley and her boyfriend Chris, both 19 years old, are transported to
the Emergency Department after being involved in a motorcycle
accident. Chris is badly hurt, but Ashley has no apparent injuries,
though she appears confused and has trouble focusing on what is
going on around her. She complains of dizziness and nausea. Her
pulse is rapid, and she is hyperventilating. The nurse should assess
Ashley's level of anxiety as:

A. mild.
B. moderate.
C. severe.
D. panic.

Correct Answer: C

Explanation/Reference:

The person whose anxiety is assessed as severe is unable to solve
problems and has a poor grasp of what's happening in his or her
environment. Somatic symptoms such as those described by Ashley
are usually present.

Vital sign changes are observed. The individual with mild anxiety might
report being mildly uncomfortable and might even find performance
enhanced. The individual with moderate anxiety grasps less
information about the situation, has some difficulty problem-solving,
and might have mild changes in vital signs. The individual in panic
demonstrates markedly disturbed behavior and might lose touch with
reality. Psychosocial Integrity

QUESTION 65

Which of the following indicates a hazard for a client on oxygen therapy?

A. A No Smoking sign is on the door.
B. The client is wearing a synthetic gown.
C. Electrical equipment is grounded.
D. Matches are removed.

Correct Answer: B

Explanation/Reference:

A synthetic gown might generate sparks of static electricity, which can be a fire hazard, particularly in the presence of oxygen. The client on oxygen therapy should wear a cotton gown. The remaining options are appropriate safety measures. Reduction of Risk Potential

QUESTION 66

When a client needs oxygen therapy, what is the highest flow rate that oxygen can be delivered via nasal cannula?

A. 2 liters/minute
B. 4 liters/minute
C. 6 liters/minute
D. 8 liters/minute

Correct Answer: C

Explanation/Reference:

The highest flow rate that oxygen can be delivered via nasal cannula is 6 liters/minute. Higher flow rates must be delivered by mask. Reduction of Risk Potential

QUESTION 67

When the nurse is determining the appropriate size of an

oropharyngeal airway to insert, what part of a client's body should she measure?

A. corner of the mouth to the tragus of the ear
B. corner of the eye to the top of the ear
C. tip of the chin to the sternum
D. tip of the nose to the earlobe

Correct Answer: A

Explanation/Reference:

An oropharyngeal airway is measured from the corner of the client's mouth, to the tragus of the ear. Reduction of Risk Potential

QUESTION 68

A nurse observes a client sitting alone and talking. When asked, the client reports that he is "talking to the voices." The nurse's next action should be:

A. touching the client to help him return to reality.
B. leaving the client alone until reality returns.
C. asking the client to describe what is happening.
D. telling the client there are no voices.

Correct Answer: C

Explanation/Reference:

Nurses might observe behavioral cues that can indicate the presence of hallucinations. Talking about the hallucinations is reassuring and validating to the client who has them. Focusing on the symptoms and asking about the hallucinations helps the client gain control. Psychosocial Integrity

A nurse observes a client sitting alone and talking. When asked, the client reports that he is "talking to the voices." The nurse's next action should be:

A. touching the client to help him return to reality.
B. leaving the client alone until reality returns.
C. asking the client to describe what is happening.
D. telling the client there are no voices.

Correct Answer: A

Explanation/Reference:

Nurses need to inform clients that there is a difference in perceptions and pay attention to the content of hallucinations. The other options are not therapeutic.Psychosocial Integrity

QUESTION 70

A 12-year-old male is brought to his primary care provider to determine whether sexual abuse has occurred. The mother states, "Because there is no permanent physical damage, he does not need any more treatment." The nurse's response should be based on which of the following pieces of information?

A. Male victims of sexual abuse seldom have long-term psychological problems.
B. Survivors of male sexual abuse might become confused about their sexual identity.
C. Unless treated, all male sex abuse survivors grow up to abuse other children.
D. All children who have been sexuallyabused have the same needs, regardless of gender.

Correct Answer: B

Explanation/Reference:

Male children are sexually abused nearly as often as female children. Perpetrators are usually men but can be women. Needs of male children who have been sexually abused might be different from the needs of female survivors. Male survivors might respond in anger, question their sexuality, use alcohol and other drugs, and might try to prove their masculinity by performing daring acts. Psychosocial Integrity.

QUESTION 71

A nurse is planning a brief treatment program for a client who was raped. A realistic, short-term goal is to:

A. identify all psychosocial problems.
B. eliminate the client's enticing behaviors.
C. resolve feelings of trauma and fear.
D. verbalize feeling about the event.

Correct Answer: D

Explanation/Reference:

A realistic short-term goal is for the client to verbalize feelings about the event. A brief treatment program is not designed to identify or resolve problems. The focus is on managing acute symptoms. If in-depth psychological problems are identified, the nurse might make referrals for treatment. Psychosocial Integrity

QUESTION 72

The intent of the Patient Self Determination Act (PSDA) of 1990 is to:

A. enhance personal control over legal care decisions.
B. encourage medical treatment decision making prior to need.
C. give one federal standard for living wills and durable powers of attorney.
D. emphasize client education.

Correct Answer: B

Explanation/Reference:

The purpose of the PSDA is to promote decision-making prior to need. Choices 1, 3 and 4 are incorrect.
The focus of the PSDA is individual health care decision-making. A federal standard for advance directives does not exist. Each state has jurisdiction regarding these policies and protocols. Coordinated Care

QUESTION 73

Client self-determination is the primary focus of:

A. malpractice insurance.
B. nursing's advocacy for clients.
C. confidentiality.
D. health care.

Correct Answer: B

Explanation/Reference:

Advocacy for clients by nurses is the primary focus of the client's right to autonomy and self- determination. Confidentiality involves the maintenance of the privacy of the client and information regarding him or her. Malpractice insurance is a type of insurance for professionals. Coordinated Care

QUESTION 74

The focus of a nurse case manager is:

A. nursing care needs at discharge.
B. the comprehensive care needs of the client for continuity of care.
C. client education needs upon discharge.
D. financial resources for needed care.

Correct Answer: B

QUESTION 75

Mr. H. is upset regarding being in the hospital for another day because he states it costs too much. The rights he is likely to demand include all of the following except:

A. the right to examine and question the bill.
B. the right to reasonable response to requests.
C. the right to refuse treatment.
D. the right to confidentiality.

Correct Answer: D

Explanation/Reference:

Confidentiality is the maintenance of privacy of information. The question does not suggest that confidentiality has been breached. The client is likely to demand the other rights and may exercise them in choosing to leave the hospital early. Coordinated Care

QUESTION 76

On first meeting, a new nurse manager makes eye contact, smiles, initiates conversation about the previous work experience of nurses, and encourages active participation by nurses in the dialogue. Her behavior is an example of:

A. aggressiveness.
B. passive aggressiveness.
C. passiveness.

D. assertiveness.

Correct Answer: D

Explanation/Reference:

This nurse manager is demonstrating assertive behavior. Aggressive behavior dominates or embarrasses. Passive behavior is nervous or timid. Passive-aggressive behavior is dominating or manipulative without directness. Coordinated Care

QUESTION 77

Legal protection of confidentiality:

A. extends only to written documentation.
B. extends to the electronic dissemination of information not identifiable to a specific client.
C. is important only within the court system.
D. extends to both written and verbal information.

Correct Answer: D

Explanation/Reference:

Legal protection of confidentiality extends to both written and verbal information identifiable as individual private health information. Coordinated Care

QUESTION 78

A 65-year-old female client is experiencing postmenopausal bleeding. Which type of physician should this client be encouraged to see?

A. a radiologist
B. a gynecologist
C. a physiatrist
D. an oncologist

Correct Answer: B

Explanation/Reference:

A gynecologist is the physician who treats and manages disease of the female reproductive organs. A radiologist evaluates X-rays. A physiatrist is the physician manager of a rehabilitation team. An oncologist treats clients with cancer. Coordinated Care

QUESTION 79

People who live in poverty are most likely to obtain health care from:
A. their primary care physician (family doctor).
B. a neighborhood clinic.
C. specialists.
D. Emergency Departments or urgent care centers.

Correct Answer: D

Explanation/Reference:

Statistical patterns of health care utilization indicate that Emergency Departments and urgent care centers provide a large portion of health care to those who live in poverty. Coordinated Care

QUESTION 80

Quality is defined as a combination of all of the following except:

A. conforming to standards.
B. performing at the minimally acceptable level.
C. meeting or exceeding customer requirements.
D. exceeding customer expectations.

Correct Answer: B

Explanation/Reference:

Compliance or performance at the minimally acceptable level is not considered quality care. Coordinated Care

QUESTION 81

All of the following are common reasons that nurses are reluctant to delegate except:

A. lack of self-confidence.
B. desire to maintain authority.
C. confidence in subordinates.
D. getting trapped in the "I can do it better myself" mindset.

Correct Answer: C

Explanation/Reference:

If a delegator has confidence in his subordinates and feels that a task will be performed correctly, he is more likely to delegate. Reasons that delegators are reluctant to delegate include their own lack of confidence, fear of losing authority or personal satisfaction, and feeling that the task can only be performed correctly if they do it themselves. Coordinated Care

QUESTION 82

Following the change of shift report, the nurse should analyze the information and set priorities accordingly. When the plan has been formulated, at what point during the shift can or should the nurse's plan be altered or modified?

A. halfway through the shift
B. at the end of the shift before the nurse reports off
C. when needs change
D. after the top-priority tasks have been completed

Correct Answer: C

Explanation/Reference:

The nurse changes the plan to respond to changes in needs. Coordinated Care

QUESTION 83

A Client states, "I eat a well-balanced diet. I do not smoke. I exercise regularly, and I have a yearly checkup with my physician. What else can I do to help prevent cancer?" The nurse should respond with which of the following statements?

A. Sleep at least 68 hours a night.
B. Practice monthly self-breast examination.
C. Reduce stress.
D. All of the above.

Correct Answer: D

Explanation/Reference:

All of the choices are methods of preventing cancer. Sleep is important in maintaining homeostasis, which helps the body respond to disease. Monthly breast examination can indicate cancer or fibrocystic disease. The body has a physiological response to stress that can decrease the immune response and increase the risk of disease. Health Promotion and Management

QUESTION 84

A 35-year-old Latin-American client wishes to lose weight to reduce her chances of developing heart disease and diabetes. The client states, "I do not know how to make my diet work with the kind of foods that my family eats." What should the nurse do first to help the client determine a suitable diet for disease prevention?

A. Provide her with copies of the approved dietary guidelines for the American Diabetic Association and the American Heart Association.
B. Ask the client to provide a list of the types of foods she eats to determine how to best meet her needs.
C. Provide a high-protein diet plan for the client.
D. Provide the client with information related to risk factors for heart disease and diabetes.

Correct Answer: B

Explanation/Reference:

Assessment is the first step. Assessing what the client eats helps the nurse determine a plan for dietary recommendations based on the ADA and AHA guidelines. Providing the client with a copy of the guidelines is important but is not the first priority. Based on the client's wish to reduce her chances of heart disease and diabetes, a high-protein diet plan might not be appropriate. Providing information to the client related to risk factors for heart disease and diabetes is important but is not the first step. Health Promotion and Management

QUESTION 85

According to the ANA Code of Ethics for Nurses, professional nurses have an ethical obligation to:

A. clients (patients).
B. the profession of nursing.
C. provide high-quality care.
D. all of the above.

Correct Answer: D

Explanation/Reference:

All the choices are elements of the ANA Code of Ethics for Nurses. Coordinated Care

QUESTION 86

The role of the incident report in risk management is:

A. liability protection.
B. to provide data for analysis by a risk manager to determine how future problems can be avoided.
C. to discipline staff for errors.
D. all of the above.

Correct Answer: B

Explanation/Reference:

Incident reports are a tool for determining how future problems can be avoided. Incident reports do not provide liability protection. Incident reports are not meant to be used for disciplining staff. Safety and Infection
Control

QUESTION 87

Which of the following individuals may legally give informed consent?

A. an 86-year-old male with advanced Alzheimer's disease
B. a 14-year-old girl needing an appendectomy who isnotan emancipated minor
C. a 72-year-old female scheduled for a heart transplant
D. a 6-month-old baby needing bowel surgery

Correct Answer: C

Explanation/Reference:

The 72-year-old client scheduled for heart transplant surgery may give informed consent for the surgery. There are no age limitations with the exception of minors. Choices 1, 2, and 4 are incorrect. An individual with advanced Alzheimer's disease is incompetent to make decisions. Only an emancipated minor may give consent (a 14-year-old child who lives alone, away from family, and is totally independent). Infants are unable to give consent. Coordinated Care

QUESTION 88

A wrong committed by one person against another (or against the property of another) that might result in a civil trial is:

A. a tort.

B. a crime.
C. a misdemeanor.
D. a felony.

Correct Answer: A

Explanation/Reference:

Torts are wrongs committed by one person against another person (or against the property of another), which might result in civil trials. A crime is also defined as a wrong against a person or their property but is considered to be against the public as well. Misdemeanors are crimes that are commonly punishable with fines or imprisonment for less than one year, with both or with parole. A felony is a serious crime punishable by imprisonment in a State or Federal penitentiary for more than one year. Coordinated Care

QUESTION 89

The family carries out its health care functions in which of the following ways?

A. Family provides very little preventive health care to its members at home.
B. Family provides sick care to its members.
C. Family pays for most health services.
D. Family decides when and where to hospitalize its members.

Correct Answer: B

Explanation/Reference:

The family provides sick care to its members. The other options are incorrect. Prevention and Early Detection of Disease

QUESTION 90

What is the primary theory that explains a family's concept of health and illness?

A. Health Belief Model
B. Education-School-Completing Factor
C. Family Health Expert Factor
D. Disconnected Family Factor

Correct Answer: A

Explanation/Reference:

The Health Belief Model describes readiness factors; the perceived feelings of susceptibility and seriousness of the health problem (the threat); and positive motivation to maintain, regain, or attain wellness. Health Promotion and Maintenance

QUESTION 91

Health promotion activities are designed to help clients:

A. reduce the risk of illness.
B. maintain maximal function.
C. promote healthy habits related to health care.
D. all of the above.

Correct Answer: D

Explanation/Reference:

Health promotion activities are designed to help clients reduce the risk of illness, maintain maximum function, and promote health habits related to health care. Health Promotion and Maintenance

QUESTION 92

Rehabilitation services begin:

A. when the client enters the health care system.
B. after the client requests rehabilitation services.
C. after the client's physical condition stabilizes.
D. when the client is discharged from the hospital.

Correct Answer: A
Explanation/Reference:

Rehabilitation services should begin when the client enters the health care system.Health Promotion and Maintenance

QUESTION 93

In conducting a health screening for 12-month-old children, the nurse expects them to have been immunized against which of the following diseases?

A. measles, polio, pertussis, hepatitis B
B. diptheria, pertussis, polio, tetanus
C. rubella, polio, pertussis, hepatitis A
D. measles, mumps, rubella, polio

Correct Answer: B

Explanation/Reference:

By 12 months of age, the child should have had DtaP and polio. MMR is not administered until a child is 12 months of age. Health Promotion and Maintenance

QUESTION 94

As part of a routine health screening, the nurse notes the play of a 2-year-old child. Which of the following is an example of age-appropriate play at this age?

A. builds towers with several blocks
B. tries to color within the lines
C. says "Mine!" when playing with toys
D. tries to jump rope

Correct Answer: C

Explanation/Reference:

Toddlers are possessive and struggle for independence. The other play activities are too advanced for a 2- year-old child.Health Promotion and Maintenance
QUESTION 95

Vaccines provide what type of immunity?

A. active
B. passive
C. transplacental
D. active and passive

Correct Answer: A

Explanation/Reference:

Vaccines provide active immunity. Passive immunity comes from antibodies produced in another human or host. Transplacental immunity comes from passive immunity transferred from mother to infant. Health Promotion and Maintenance

QUESTION 96

A 2-year-old child diagnosed with HIV comes to a clinic for immunizations. Which of the following vaccines should the nurse expect to administer in addition to the scheduled vaccines?

A. pneumococcal vaccine
B. hepatitis A vaccine
C. Lyme disease vaccine
D. typhoid vaccine

Correct Answer: A

Explanation/Reference:

Pneumococcal vaccine should be administered as a supplemental vaccine. Hepatitis A vaccine is for travelers and individuals with chronic liver disease. The Lyme disease vaccine is for people between the ages of 15 and 70 who are at risk for Lyme disease (transmitted by ticks primarily). The typhoid vaccine is for workers in microbiology laboratories who frequently work with Salmonella typhi. Health Promotion and Maintenance

QUESTION 97

Ms. Petty is having difficulty falling asleep. Which of the following measures promote sleep?

A. exercising vigorously for 20 minutes each night beginning at 9:30 p.m.
B. taking a cool shower and drinking a hot cup of tea
C. watching TV nightly until midnight
D. getting a back rub and drinking a glass of warm milk

Correct Answer: D

Explanation/Reference:

These are appropriate measure to promote sleep. Choices 1, 2, and 3 are all stimulation actions that increase arousal and wakefulness. Basic Care and Comfort

QUESTION 98

A 4-year-old client is unable to go to sleep at night in the hospital. Which nursing intervention best promotes sleep for the child?

A. turning out the room light and closing the door
B. tiring the child during the evening with play exercises
C. identifying the child's home bedtime rituals and following them
D. encouraging visitation by friends during the evening

Correct Answer: C

Explanation/Reference:

Preschool-age children require bedtime rituals that should be followed in the hospital if possible.
Choice 1 increases a child's fear. Choices 2 and 4 do not promote sleep. Basic Care and Comfort

QUESTION 99

The 24-hour day-night cycle is known as:

A. circadian rhythm.
B. infradium rhythm.
C. ultradian rhythm.
D. non-REM rhythm.

Correct Answer: A

Explanation/Reference:

Circadian rhythm is rhythmic repetition of patterns each 24 hours. The other options are incorrect.Basic Care and Comfort

QUESTION 100

Which of the following solutions is routinely used to flush an IV device before and after the administration of blood to a client?

A. 0.9% sodium chloride
B. 5% dextrose in water solution
C. sterile water
D. Heparin sodium

Correct Answer: A

Explanation/Reference:

Normal saline is 0.9% sodium chloride. This solution has the same osmolarity as blood. Its use does not cause lysis of cells. Choices 2 and 3 are hypotonic solutions that can cause cell lysis. Choice 4 is an anticoagulant. Pharmacological Therapies

QUESTION 101

Central venous access devices (CVADs) are frequently utilized to administer chemotherapy. What is an advantage of using CVADs for chemotherapeutic agent administration?

A. CVADs are less expensive than a peripheral IV.
B. Weekly administration is possible.
C. Chemotherapeutic agents can be caustic to smaller veins.
D. The client or family can administer the drug at home.

Correct Answer: C

Explanation/Reference:

Many chemotherapeutic drugs are vesicants (highly active corrosive materials that can produce tissue damage even in low concentrations). Administration into a large vein is optimal. Choice 1 is incorrect because CVADs are more expensive than a peripheral IV. Choice 2 is incorrect because dosing depends on the drug.
Choice 4 is incorrect because IV chemotherapeutic agents are not routinely administered at home; they are usually given in a hospital or in an outpatient or clinic setting. Pharmacological Therapies

QUESTION 102

The chemotherapeutic DNA alkylating agents such as nitrogen
mustards are effective because they:

A. cross-link DNA strands with covalent bonds between alkyl groups
   on the drug and guanine bases on DNA.
B. have few, if any, side effects.
C. are used to treat multiple types of cancer.
D. are cell-cycle-specific agents.

Correct Answer: A

Explanation/Reference:

Alkylating agents are highly reactive chemicals that introduce alkyl
radicals into biologically active molecules and thereby prevent their
proper functioning, replication, and transcription. Choice 2 is incorrect
because alkylating agents have numerous side effects including
alopecia, nausea, vomiting, and myelosuppression.

Choice 3 is incorrect because nitrogen mustards have a broad
spectrum of activity against chronic lymphocytic leukemia, non-
Hodgkin's lymphoma, and breast and ovarian cancer, but they are
effective chemotherapeutic agents because of DNA crosslinkage.
Choice 4 is incorrect because alkylating agents are non-cell-cycle-
specific agents. Pharmacological Therapies

QUESTION 103

Medication bound to protein can have which of the following effects?

A. enhancement of drug availability
B. rapid distribution of the drug to receptor sites
C. less availability to produce desired medicinal effects
D. increased metabolism of the drug by the liver

Correct Answer: C

Explanation/Reference:

Only an unbound drug can be distributed to active receptor sites. Therefore, the more of a drug that is bound to protein, the less it is available for the desired drug effect. Choice 1 is incorrect because less drug is available if it is bound to protein. Choice 2 is incorrect because distribution to receptor sites is irrelevant if the drug, which is bound to protein, cannot bind with a receptor site. Choice 4 is incorrect because metabolism is not increased. The liver first has to remove the drug from the protein molecule before metabolism can occur. The protein is then free to return to circulation and be used again. Pharmacological Therapies

QUESTION 104

The physician orders the antibiotics ampicillin (Omnipen) and gentamicin (Garamycin) for a newly admitted client with an infection. The nurse should:

A. administer both medications simultaneously.
B. give the medications sequentially, and flush well between them.
C. ask the physician or pharmacy which medication to give first and how long to wait before giving the other drug.
D. start one medication now and begin the other medication in 24 hours.

Correct Answer: B

Explanation/Reference:

A client with an infection needs both antibiotics as soon a possible. However, the pH of ampicillin is 8 10, and the pH of gentamicin is 35.5 (making them incompatible when given together). Flushing well between drugs is necessary. Choice 3 is incorrect because the PN determines the correct steps and consults with the pharmacist and the physician as necessary. Choice 4 is incorrect because delaying the second medication by several hours slows the treatment of the client's infection. Pharmacological Therapies

QUESTION 105

Fat emulsions are frequently administered as a part of total parenteral nutrition. Which statement is true regarding fat emulsions?

A. They have a high energy-to-fluid-volume ratio.
B. Even though hypertonic, they are well tolerated.
C. They are a basic solution secondary to the addition of sodium hydroxide (NaOH).
D. The pH is alkaline, making them compatible with most medications.

Correct Answer: A

Explanation/Reference:

They have a high energy-to-fluid-volume ratio. Fat emulsions are formulated in 10%, 20%, and 30% solutions and supply 1.1, 2, and 3 kilocalories respectively for each milliliter. A milliliter of 5% dextrose only supplies 0.17 kilocalories. Choices 2, 3, and 4 are incorrect because fat emulsions are essentially pH neutral and isotonic. Pharmacological Therapies

QUESTION 106

The nurse wishes to decrease a client's use of denial and increase the client's expression of feelings. To do this the nurse should:

A. tell the client to stop using the defense mechanism of denial.
B. positively reinforce each expression of feelings.
C. instruct the client to express feelings.
D. challenge the client each time denial is used.

Correct Answer: B

Explanation/Reference:

The nurse should positively reinforce each expression of feelings. Psychosocial Integrity

QUESTION 107

A 57-year-old woman is recently widowed. She states, "I will never be able to learn how to manage the finances. My husband did all of that." Select the nurse's response that could help raise the client's self-esteem.

A. "You feel inadequate because you have never learned to balance a checkbook."
B. "You should have insisted your husband teach you about the finances."
C. "You are strong and will learn how to manage your finances after awhile."
D. "Why don't you take a class in basic finance from the local college?"

Correct Answer: C

Explanation/Reference:

The nurse can raise the client's self-esteem by communicating confidence the client can participate in actively finding solutions to the problem. The nurse also conveys the client is a worthwhile person by listening and accepting the client's feelings and praising the client for seeking assistance. Psychosocial Integrity

QUESTION 108

An elderly client denies that abuse is occurring. Which of the following factors could be a barrier for the client to admit being a victim?

A. knowledge that elder abuse is rare
B. personal belief that abuse is deserved
C. lack of developmentally appropriate screening tools
D. fear of reprisal or further violence if the incident is reported

Correct Answer: D

Explanation/Reference:

Barriers to reporting elder abuse include victim shame, fear of reprisals, fear of loss of caregiver, and lack of knowledge of agencies that provide services. Many elders fear that reporting abuse results in their placement in long-term care because the current caregiver is the abuser. Choices 1 and 3 are incorrect. Choice 2 might be true but is not the best choice. Psychosocial Integrity

QUESTION 109

The nurse observes bilateral bruises on the arms of an elderly client in a long-term care facility. Which of the following questions should the nurse ask this client?

A. "How did you get those bruises?"
B. "Did someone grab you by your arms?"
C. "Do you fall often?"
D. "What did you bump against?"

Correct Answer: B

Explanation/Reference:

Using a direct approach is best when asking about suspected abuse. Clients are reluctant to report abuse because of shame and fear of reprisal. Psychosocial Integrity

QUESTION 110

Distribution of a drug to various tissues is dependent on the amount of cardiac output to each type of tissue. Which tissue would receive the highest amount of cardiac output and thus the highest amount of a drug?

A. skin
B. adipose tissue
C. skeletal muscle
D. myocardium

Correct Answer: D

Explanation/Reference:

Highly perfused tissue includes all vital organs: the brain, heart, kidneys, adrenal glands, and liver. Choices 1, 2, and 3 are incorrect because the skin and adipose tissue are poorly perfused, while the skeletal muscle is better perfused. Pharmacological Therapies

QUESTION 111

A syringe pump is a type of electronic infusion pump used to infuse fluids or medications directly from a syringe. This device is commonly used for:

A. solutions administered in obstetrics.
B. dilute antibiotics.
C. large volumes of IV solution.
D. the neonatal and pediatric populations.

Correct Answer: D

Explanation/Reference:

Small volumes of medication or fluids are delivered and sometimes at slow rates to neonates and pediatric clients. The syringe pump allows precise infusion of small volumes. Choice 1 is incorrect because a syringe pump can be used in almost any setting, but is not generally for adult clients. Choices 2 and 3 are incorrect because large volumes of fluids are not administered with a syringe pump. Pharmacological Therapies

QUESTION 112

A client with massive chest and head injuries is admitted to the ICU from the Emergency Department. All of the following are true except:

A. a declaration of wishes or documentation of wishes regarding organ donation by the donor is necessary for organ harvesting.
B. the physician in charge of the case is the only person allowed to decide whether organ donation can occur.
C. the client's legally responsible party may make the decision for organ donation for the donor if the client is unable to do so.
D. the organ procurement organization makes the decision regarding which organs to harvest.

Correct Answer: C

Explanation/Reference:

The client's legally responsible party may make the decision for organ donation if the client is unable to do so.
The donor (or legally responsible party for the donor), the physician, and the organ-procurement organization are all involved in the process regarding whether organ donation is appropriate for a specific donor.
Coordinated Care

QUESTION 113

A 45-year-old client with type I diabetes is in need of support services upon discharge from a skilled rehabilitation unit. Which of the following services is an example of a skilled support service?

A. shopping for groceries
B. house cleaning
C. transportation to physician's visits
D. medication instruction

Correct Answer: D

Explanation/Reference:

The only skilled service listed is medication instruction. Grocery shopping, house-cleaning services, and transportation services are all examples of unskilled services offered by volunteer and fee-for-service agencies. Coordinated Care

QUESTION 114

Narrow therapeutic index medications:

A. are drug formulations with limited pharmacokinetic variability.
B. have limited value and require no monitoring of blood levels.
C. have less than a twofold difference in minimum toxic levels and minimum effective concentration in the blood.
D. have limited potency and side effects.

Correct Answer: C

Explanation/Reference:

The therapeutic index is the ratio between the median lethal dose and median effective dose of a drug.

It provides a general indication of the margin of safety of a drug. Choice 1 is incorrect because pharmacokinetics is the process of adsorption, distribution, metabolism, and elimination. Choice 2 is incorrect because narrow therapeutic index drugs require close monitoring since there is often little difference between the desired drug effect and toxicity.

Choice 4 is incorrect because narrow therapeutic index drugs have the potential for severe toxic effects with only slight increases in the dose or slight decreases in elimination. Pharmacological Therapies

QUESTION 115

A client can receive the mumps, measles, rubella (MMR) vaccine if he or she:

A. is pregnant.
B. is immunocompromised.
C. is allergic to neomycin.
D. has a cold.

Correct Answer: D

Explanation/Reference:

A simple cold without fever does not preclude vaccination. Choices 1 and 2 are incorrect because pregnant women and immunocompromised individuals cannot have the MMR vaccine because the rubella component is a live virus and might cause birth defects and/or disease.

Choice 3 is incorrect because the American Academy of Pediatrics states, "Persons who have experienced anaphylactic reactions to topically or systemically administered neomycin should not receive measles vaccine."

Pharmacological Therapies

QUESTION 116

A chemical reaction between drugs prior to their administration or absorption is known as:

A. a drug incompatibility.
B. a side effect.
C. an adverse event.
D. an allergic response.

Correct Answer: A

Explanation/Reference:

This occurs most often when drug solutions are combined before they are given intravenously but can occur with orally administered drugs as well. Choices 2, 3, and 4 are incorrect because drugs can cause these events after administration and absorption. Pharmacological Therapies

QUESTION 117

A client is given an opiate drug for pain relief following general anesthesia. The client becomes extremely somnolent with respiratory depression. The physician is likely to order the administration of:

A. naloxone (Narcan).
B. labetalol (Normodyne).
C. neostigmine (Prostigmin).
D. thiothixene (Navane).

Correct Answer: A

Explanation/Reference:

Naloxone is an opiate antagonist. It attaches to opiate receptors and blocks or reverses the action of narcotic analgesics. Choice 2 is

incorrect because Labetalol is a beta blocker. Choice 3 is incorrect because Neostigmine is an anticholinesterase agent. Choice 4 is incorrect because Thiothixene is an antipsychotic agent.
Pharmacological
Therapies

QUESTION 118

A 25-year-old client believes she may be pregnant with her first child. She schedules an obstetric examination with the nurse practitioner to determine the status of her possible pregnancy. Her last menstrual period began May 20, and her estimated date of confinement using Nägele's rule is:

A. March 27
B. February 1
C. February 27
D. January 3

Correct Answer: C

Explanation/Reference:

(A)March 27 is a miscalculation. (B) February 1 is a miscalculation. (C) February 27 is the correct answer. To calculate the estimated date of confinement using Nagele's rule, subtract 3 months from the date that the last menstrual cycle began and then add 7 days to the result. (D) January 3 is a miscalculation.

QUESTION 119

The nurse practitioner determines that a client is approximately 9 weeks' gestation. During the visit, the practitioner informs the client about symptoms of physical changes that she will experience during her first trimester, such as:

A. Nausea and vomiting
B. Quickening

C. A 68 lb weight gain

D. Abdominal enlargement

Correct Answer: A

Explanation/Reference:

(A) Nausea and vomiting are experienced by almost half of all pregnant women during the first 3 months of pregnancy as a result of elevated human chorionic gonadotropin levels and changed carbohydrate metabolism.

(B) Quickening is the mother's perception of fetal movement and generally does not occur until 1820 weeks after the last menstrual period in primigravidas, but it may occur as early as 16 weeks in multigravidas.

(C) During the first trimester there should be only a modest weight gain of 24 lb. It is not uncommon for women to lose weight during the first trimester owing to nausea and/or vomiting. (D) Physical changes are not apparent until the second trimester, when the uterus rises out of the pelvis.

QUESTION 120

A client is 6 weeks pregnant. During her first prenatal visit, she asks, "How much alcohol is safe to drink during pregnancy?" The nurse's response is:

A. Up to 1 oz daily

B. Up to 2 oz daily

C. Up to 4 oz weekly

D. No alcohol

Correct Answer: D

Explanation/Reference:

(A, B, C) No amount of alcohol has been determined safe for pregnant women. Alcohol should be avoided owing to the risk of fetal alcohol syndrome. (D) The recommended safe dosage of alcohol consumption during pregnancy is none.

QUESTION 121

A 38-year-old pregnant woman visits her nurse practitioner for her regular prenatal checkup. She is 30 weeks' gestation. The nurse should be alert to which condition related to her age?

A. Iron-deficiency anemia
B. Sexually transmitted disease (STD)
C. Intrauterine growth retardation
D. Pregnancy-induced hypertension (PIH)

Correct Answer: D

Explanation/Reference:

(A) Iron-deficiency anemia can occur throughout pregnancy and is not age related.
(B) STDs can occur prior to or during pregnancy and are not age related.
(C) Intrauterine growth retardation is an abnormal process where fetal development and maturation are delayed. It is not age related.
(D) Physical risks for the pregnant client older than 35 include increased risk for PIH, cesarean delivery, fetal and neonatal mortality, and trisomy.

QUESTION 122

A client returns for her 6-month prenatal checkup and has gained 10 lb in 2 months. The results of her physical examination are normal. How does the nurse interpret the effectiveness of the instruction about diet and weight control?

A. She is compliant with her diet as previously taught.
B. She needs further instruction and reinforcement.
C. She needs to increase her caloric intake.
D. She needs to be placed on a restrictive diet immediately.

Correct Answer: B

(A) She is probably not compliant with her diet and exercise program. Recommended weight gain during second and third trimesters is approximately 12 lb.
(B) Because of her excessive weight gain of 10 lb in 2 months, she needs re-evaluation of her eating habits and reinforcement of proper dietary habits for pregnancy. A 2200-calorie diet is recommended for most pregnant women with a weight gain of 2730 lb over the 9-month period. With rapid and excessive weight gain, PIH should also be suspected.
(C) She does not need to increase her caloric intake, but she does need to re-evaluate dietary habits. Ten pounds in 2 months is excessive weight gain during pregnancy, and health teaching is warranted.
(D) Restrictive dieting is not recommended during pregnancy.

QUESTION 123

Pregnant women with diabetes often have problems related to the effectiveness of insulin in controlling their glucose levels during their second half of pregnancy. The nurse teaches the client that this is due to:

A. Decreased glomerular filtration and increased tubular absorption
B. Decreased estrogen levels
C. Decreased progesterone levels
D. Increased human placental lactogen levels

Correct Answer: D

Explanation/Reference:

(A) There is a rise in glomerular filtration rate in the kidneys in conjunction with decreased tubular glucose reabsorption, resulting in glycosuria.
(B) Insulin is inhibited by increased levels of estrogen.
(C) Insulin is inhibited by increased levels of progesterone.
(D) Human placental lactogen levels increase later in pregnancy. This

hormonal antagonist reduces insulin's effectiveness, stimulates
lipolysis, and increases the circulation of free fatty acids.

QUESTION 124

Diabetes during pregnancy requires tight metabolic control of glucose
levels to prevent perinatal mortality. When evaluating the pregnant
client, the nurse knows the recommended serum glucose range during
pregnancy is:

A. 70 mg/dL and 120 mg/dL
B. 100 mg/dL and 200 mg/dL
C. 40 mg/dL and 130 mg/dL
D. 90 mg/dL and 200 mg/dL

Correct Answer: A

Explanation/Reference:

(A) The recommended range is 70120 mg/dL to reduce the risk of
perinatal mortality. (B, C, D) These levels are not recommended. The
higher the blood glucose, the worse the prognosis for the fetus.
Hypoglycemia can also have detrimental effects on the fetus.

QUESTION 125

When assessing fetal heart rate status during labor, the monitor
displays late decelerations with tachycardia and decreasing variability.
What action should the nurse take?

A. Continue monitoring because this is a normal occurrence.
B. Turn client on right side.
C. Decrease IV fluids.
D. Report to physician or midwife.

Correct Answer: D

Explanation/Reference:

(A) This is not a normal occurrence. Late decelerations need prompt
intervention for immediate infant recovery.

(B) To increase O2 perfusion to the unborn infant, the mother should be placed on her left side.
(C) IV fluids should be increased, not decreased.
(D) Immediate action is warranted, such as reporting findings, turning mother on left side, administering O2, discontinuing oxytocin (Pitocin), assessing maternal blood pressure and the labor process, preparing for immediate cesarean delivery, and explaining plan of action to client.

QUESTION 126

A client has been diagnosed as being preeclamptic. The physician orders magnesium sulfate. Magnesium sulfate (MgSO4) is used in the management of preeclampsia for:

A. Prevention of seizures

B. Prevention of uterine contractions

C. Sedation

D. Fetal lung protection

Correct Answer: A

Explanation/Reference:

(A) MgSO4 is classified as an anticonvulsant drug. In preeclampsia management, MgSO4 is used for prevention of seizures.
(B) MgSO4 has been used to inhibit hyperactive labor, but results are questionable.

(C) Negative side effects such as respiratory depression should not be confused with generalized sedation.
(D) MgSO4 does not affect lung maturity. The infant should be assessed for neuromuscular and respiratory depression.

QUESTION 127

The predominant purpose of the first Apgar scoring of a newborn is to:

A. Determine gross abnormal motor function

B. Obtain a baseline for comparison with the infant's future adaptation to the environment

C. Evaluate the infant's vital functions

D. Determine the extent of congenital malformations

Correct Answer: C

Explanation/Reference:

(A) Apgar scores are not related to the infant's care, but to the infant's physical condition.
(B) Apgar scores assess the current physical condition of the infant and are not related to future environmental adaptation.
(C) The purpose of the Apgar system is to evaluate the physical condition of the newborn at birth and to determine if there is an immediate need for resuscitation.
(D) Congenital malformations are not one of the areas assessed with Apgar scores.

QUESTION 128

Provide the 1-minute Apgar score for an infant born with the following findings: Heart rate: Above 100 Respiratory effort: Slow, irregular Muscle tone: Some flexion of extremities Reflex irritability: Vigorous cry Color: Body pink, blue extremities

A. 7
B. 10
C. 8
D. 9

Correct Answer: A

Explanation/Reference:

(A) Seven out of a possible perfect score of 10 is correct. Two points are given for heart rate above 100; 1 point is given for slow, irregular respiratory effort; 1 point is given for some flex- ion of extremities in assessing muscle tone; 2 points are given for vigorous cry in assessing reflex irritability; 1 point is assessed for color when the body is pink with blue extremities (acrocyanosis).
(B) For a perfect Apgar score of 10, the infant would have a heart rate over 100 but would also have a good cry, active motion, and be

completely pink.
(C) For an Apgar score of 8 the respiratory rate, muscle tone, or color
would need to fall into the 2-point rather than the 1-point category.
(D) For this infant to receive an Apgar score of 9, four of the areas
evaluated would need ratings of 2 points and one area, a rating of 1
point.

QUESTION 129

A pregnant woman at 36 weeks' gestation is followed for PIH and
develops proteinuria. To increase protein in her diet, which of the
following foods will provide the greatest amount of protein when added
to her intake of 100 mL of milk?

A. Fifty milliliters light cream and 2 tbsp corn syrup
B. Thirty grams powdered skim milk and 1 egg
C. One small scoop (90 g) vanilla ice cream and 1 tbsp chocolate
   syrup
D. One package vitamin-fortified gelatin drink

Correct Answer: B

Explanation/Reference:

(A) This choice would provide more unwanted fat and sugar than
protein.
(B) Skim milk would add protein. Eggs are good sources of protein
while low in fat and calories.
(C) The benefit of protein from ice cream would be outweighed by the
fat content. Chocolate syrup has caffeine, which is contraindicated or
limited in pregnancy.
(D) Although most animal proteins are higher in protein than plant
proteins, gelatin is not. It loses protein during the processing for food
consumption.

QUESTION 130

The physician recommends immediate hospital admission for a client
with PIH. She says to the nurse, "It's not so easy for me to just go right
to the hospital like that." After acknowledging her feelings, which of
these approaches by the nurse would probably be best?

A. Stress to the client that her husband would want her to do what is best for her health.
B. Explore with the client her perceptions of why she is unable to go to the hospital.
C. Repeat the physician's reasons for advising immediate hospitalization.
D. Explain to the client that she is ultimately responsible for her own welfare and that of her baby.

Correct Answer: B

Explanation/Reference:

(A) This answer does not hold the client accountable for her own health.
(B) The nurse should explore potential reasons for the client's anxiety: are there small children at home, is the husband out of town? The nurse should aid the client in seeking support or interventions to decrease the anxiety of hospitalization.
(C) Repeating the physician's reason for recommending hospitalization may not aid the client in dealing with her reasons for anxiety.
 (D) The concern for self and welfare of baby may be secondary to a woman who is in a crisis situation. The nurse should explore the client's potential reasons for anxiety. For example, is there another child in the home who is ill, or is there a husband who is overseas and not able to return on short notice?

QUESTION 131

Which of the following findings would be abnormal in a postpartal woman?

A. Chills shortly after delivery
B. Pulse rate of 60 bpm in morning on first postdelivery day
C. Urinary output of 3000 mL on the second day after delivery
D. An oral temperature of 101F (38.3C) on the third day after delivery

Correct Answer: D

Explanation/Reference:

(A) Frequently the mother experiences a shaking chill immediately after delivery, which is related to a nervous response or to vasomotor changes. If not followed by a fever, it is clinically innocuous.

(B) The pulse rate during the immediate postpartal period may be low but presents no cause for alarm. The body attempts to adapt to the decreased pressures intra-abdominally as wellas from the reduction of blood flow to the vascular bed.

(C) Urinary output increases during the early postpartal period (1224 hours) owing to diuresis. The kidneys must eliminate an estimated 20003000 mL of extracellular fluid associated with a normal pregnancy.

(D) A temperature of 100.4F (38C) may occur after delivery as a result of exertion and dehydration of labor. However, any temperature greater than 100.4F needs further investigation to identify any infectious process.

QUESTION 132

What is the most effective method to identify early breast cancer lumps?

A. Mammograms every 3 years
B. Yearly checkups performed by physician
C. Ultrasounds every 3 years
D. Monthly breast self-examination

Correct Answer: D

Explanation/Reference:

(A) Mammograms are less effective than breast self-examination for the diagnosis of abnormalities in younger women, who have denser breast tissue. They are more effective for women older than 40.
(B) Up to 15% of early-stage breast cancers are detected by physical examination; however, 95% are detected by women doing breast self-examination.
(C) Ultrasound is used primarily to determine the location of cysts and to distinguish cysts from solid masses.
(D) Monthly breast self-examination has been shown to be the most effective method for early detection of breast cancer. Approximately 95% of lumps are detected by women themselves.

QUESTION 133

Which of the following risk factors associated with breast cancer would a nurse consider most significant in a client's history?

A. Menarche after age 13
B. Nulliparity
C. Maternal family history of breast cancer
D. Early menopause

Correct Answer: C

Explanation/Reference:

(A) Women who begin menarche late (after 13 years old) have a lower risk of developing breast cancer than women who have begun earlier. Average age for menarche is 12.5 years.
(B) Women who have never been pregnant have an increased risk for breast cancer, but a positive family history poses an even greater risk.
(C) A positive family history puts a woman at an increased risk of developing breast cancer. It is recommended that mammography screening begin 5 years before the age at which an immediate female relative was diagnosed with breast cancer.
(D) Early menopause decreases the risk of developing breast cancer.

QUESTION 134

Which of the following procedures is necessary to establish a definitive diagnosis of breast cancer?

A. Diaphanography
B. Mammography
C. Thermography
D. Breast tissue biopsy

Correct Answer: D

Explanation/Reference:

(A) Diaphanography, also known as transillumination, is a painless,

noninvasive imaging technique that involves shining a light source through the breast tissue to visualize the interior. It must be used in conjunction with a mammogram and physical examination.
(B) Mammography is a useful tool for screening but is not considered a means of diagnosing breast cancers.

(C) Thermography is a pictorial representation of heat patterns on the surface of the breast. Breast cancers appear as a "hot spot" owing to their higher metabolic rate.
(D) Biopsy either by needleaspiration or by surgical incision is the primary diagnostic technique for confirming the presence of cancer cells.

QUESTION 135

The nurse should know that according to current thinking, the most important prognostic factor for a client with breast cancer is:

A. Tumor size
B. Axillary node status
C. Client's previous history of disease
D. Client's level of estrogen-progesterone receptor assays

Correct Answer: B

Explanation/Reference:

(A) Although tumor size is a factor in classification of cancer growth, it is not an indicator of lymph node spread.
(B) Axillary node status is the most important indicator for predicting how far the cancer has spread. If the lymph nodes are positive for cancer cells, the prognosis is poorer.
 (C) The client's previous history of cancer puts her at an increased risk for breast cancer recurrence, especially if the cancer occurred in the other breast. It does not predict prognosis, however.
 (D) The estrogen- progesterone assay test is used to identify present tumors being fed from an estrogen site within the body. Some breast cancers grow rapidly as long as there is an estrogen supply such as from the ovaries. The estrogen- progesterone assay test does not indicate the prognosis.

QUESTION 136

When teaching a sex education class, the nurse identifies the most common STDs in the United States as:

A. Chlamydia
B. Herpes genitalis
C. Syphilis
D. Gonorrhea

Correct Answer: A
Explanation/Reference:

(A) Chlamydia trachomatis infection is the most common STD in the United States. The Centers for Disease Control and Prevention recommend screening of all high-risk women, such as adolescents and women with multiple sex partners.

(B) Herpes simplex genitalia is estimated to be found in 520 million people in the United States and is rising in occurrence yearly.

(C) Syphilis is a chronic infection caused by Treponema pallidum. Over the last several years the number of people infected has begun to increase.

(D) Gonorrhea is a bacterial infection caused by the organism Neisseria gonorrhea. Although gonorrhea is common, chlamydia is still the most common STD.

QUESTION 137

A 30-year-old male client is admitted to the psychiatric unit with a diagnosis of bipolar disorder. For the last 2 months, his family describes him as being "on the move," sleeping 34 hours nightly, spending lots of money, and losing approximately 10 lb. During the initial assessment with the client, the nurse would expect him to exhibit which of the following?

A. Short, polite responses to interview questions
B. Introspection related to his present situation
C. Exaggerated self-importance
D. Feelings of helplessness and hopelessness

Correct Answer: C

Explanation/Reference:

(A) During the manic phase of bipolar disorder, clients have short
attention spans and may be abusive toward authority figures.
(B) Introspection requires focusing and concentration; clients with
mania experience flight of ideas, which prevents concentration.
(C) Grandiosity and an inflated sense of self-worth are characteristic of
this disorder.
(D) Feelings of helplessness and hopelessness are symptoms of the
depressive stage of bipolar disorder.

QUESTION 138

The therapeutic blood-level range for lithium is:

A. 0.251.0 mEq/L
B. 0.51.5 mEq/L
C. 1.02.0 mEq/L
D. 2.02.5 mEq/L

Correct Answer: B

Explanation/Reference:

(A) This range is too low to be therapeutic.
(B) This is the therapeutic range for lithium.
 (C) This range is above the therapeutic level.
(D) This range is toxic and may cause severe side effects.

QUESTION 139

A client with bipolar disorder taking lithium tells the nurse that he has
ringing in his ears, blurred vision, and diarrhea. The nurse notices a
slight tremor in his left hand and a slurring pattern to his speech. Which
of the following actions by the nurse is appropriate?

A. Administer a stat dose of lithium as necessary.
B. Recognize this as an expected response to lithium.
C. Request an order for a stat blood lithium level.
D. Give an oral dose of lithium antidote.

Correct Answer: C

Explanation/Reference:

(A) These symptoms are indicative of lithium toxicity. A stat dose of lithium could be fatal.
(B) These are toxic effects of lithium therapy.
(C) The client is exhibiting symptoms of lithium toxicity, which may be validated by lab studies.
(D) There is no known lithium antidote.

QUESTION 140

Which of the following activities would be most appropriate during occupational therapy for a client with bipolar disorder?

A. Playing cards with other clients
B. Working crossword puzzles
C. Playing tennis with a staff member
D. Sewing beads on a leather belt

Correct Answer: C

Explanation/Reference:

(A) This activity is too competitive, and the manic client might become abusive toward the other clients.
(B) During mania, the client's attention span is too short to accomplish this task.
(C) This activity uses gross motor skills, eases tension, and expands excess energy. A staff member is better equipped to interact therapeutically with clients.
(D) This activity requires the use of fine motor skills and is very tedious.

QUESTION 141

A client diagnosed with bipolar disorder continues to be hyperactive and to lose weight. Which of the following nutritional interventions would be most therapeutic for him at this time?

A. Small, frequent feedings of foods that can be carried
B. Tube feedings with nutritional supplements
C. Allowing him to eat when and what he wants
D. Giving him a quiet place where he can sit down to eat meals

Correct Answer: A

Explanation/Reference:

(A) The manic client is unable to sit still long enough to eat an adequate meal. Small, frequent feedings with finger foods allow him to eat during periods of activity.
(B) This type of therapy should be implemented when other methods have been exhausted.

(C) The manic client should not be in control of his treatment plan. This type of client may forget to eat.
(D) The manic client is unable to sit down to eat full meals.

QUESTION 142

Three weeks following discharge, a male client is readmitted to the psychiatric unit for depression. His wife stated that he had threatened to kill himself with a handgun. As the nurse admits him to the unit, he says, "I wish I were dead because I am worthless to everyone; I guess I am just no good." Which response by the nurse is most appropriate at this time?

A. "I don't think you are worthless. I'm glad to see you, and we will help you."
B. "Don't you think this is a sign of your illness?"
C. "I know with your wife and new baby that you do have a lot to live for."
D. "You've been feeling sad and alone for some time now?"

Correct Answer: D

Explanation/Reference:

(A) This response does not acknowledge the client's feelings.
 (B) This is a closed question and does not encourage communication.
(C) This response negates the client's feelings and does not require a
response from the client.
 (D) This acknowledges the client's implied thoughts and feelings and
encourages a response.

QUESTION 143

Which of the following statements relevant to a suicidal client is
correct?

A. The more specific a client's plan, the more likely he or she is to
   attempt suicide.
B. A client who is unsuccessful at a first suicide attempt is not likely to
   make future attempts.
C. A client who threatens suicide is just seeking attention and is not
   likely to attempt suicide.
D. Nurses who care for a client who has attempted suicide should not
   make any reference to the word "suicide" in order to protect the
   client's ego.

Correct Answer: A
Explanation/Reference:

(A) This is a high-risk factor for potential suicide.
(B) A previous suicide attempt is a definite risk factor for subsequent
attempts.
(C) Every threat of suicide should be taken seriously.
 (D) The client should be asked directly about his or her intent to do
bodily harm. The client is never hurt by direct, respectful questions.

QUESTION 144

The physician orders fluoxetine (Prozac) for a depressed client. Which
of the following should the nurse remember about fluoxetine?

A. Because fluoxetine is a tricyclic antidepressant, it may precipitate a
   hypertensive crisis.
B. The therapeutic effect of the drug occurs 24 weeks after treatment
   is begun.

C. Foods such as aged cheese, yogurt, soy sauce, and bananas
should not be eaten with this drug.
D. Fluoxetine may be administered safely in combination with
monoamine oxidase (MAO) inhibitors.

Correct Answer: B

Explanation/Reference:

(A) Fluoxetine is not a tricyclic antidepressant. It is an atypical
antidepressant.
 (B) This statement is true.
(C) These foods are high in tyramine and should be avoided when the
client is taking MAO inhibitors. Fluoxetine is not an MAO inhibitor.
(D) Fatal reactions have been reported in clients receiving fluoxetine in
combination with MAO inhibitors.

QUESTION 145

The day following his admission, the nurse sits down by a male client
on the sofa in the dayroom. He was admitted for depression and
thoughts of suicide. He looks at the nurse and says, "My life is so bad
no one can do anything to help me." The most helpful initial response
by the nurse would be:

A. "It concerns me that you feel so badly when you have so many
positive things in your life."

B. "It will take a few weeks for you to feel better, so you need to be
patient."
C. "You are telling me that you are feeling hopeless at this point?"
D. "Let's play cards with some of the other clients to get your mind off
your problems for now."

Correct Answer: C

Explanation/Reference:

(A) This response does not acknowledge the client's feelings and may
increase his feelings of guilt.
(B) This response denotes false reassurance.

(C) This response acknowledges the client's feelings and invites a response.
(D) This response changes the subject and does not allow the client to talk about his feelings.

QUESTION 146

A long-term goal for the nurse in planning care for a depressed, suicidal client would be to:

A. Provide him with a safe and structured environment.

B. Assist him to develop more effective coping mechanisms.

C. Have him sign a "no-suicide" contract.

D. Isolate him from stressful situations that may precipitate a depressive episode.

Correct Answer: B

Explanation/Reference:

(A) This statement represents a short-term goal.
 (B) Long-term therapy should be directed toward assisting the client to cope effectively with stress.
(C) Suicide contracts represent short-term interventions.
(D) This statement represents an unrealistic goal. Stressful situations cannot be avoided in reality.

QUESTION 147

After 3 weeks of treatment, a severely depressed client suddenly begins to feel better and starts interacting appropriately with other clients and staff. The nurse knows that this client has an increased risk for:

A. Suicide

B. Exacerbation of depressive symptoms

C. Violence toward others

D. Psychotic behavior

Correct Answer: A

Explanation/Reference:

(A) When the severely depressed client suddenly begins to feel better, it often indicates that the client has made the decision to kill himself or herself and has developed a plan to do so.
(B) Improvement in behavior is not indicative of an exacerbation of depressive symptoms.
(C) The depressed client has a tendency for self-violence, not violence toward others.
 (D) Depressive behavior is not always accompanied by psychotic behavior.

QUESTION 148

Nursing care for the substance abuse client experiencing alcohol withdrawal delirium includes:

A. Maintaining seizure precautions
B. Restricting fluid intake
C. Increasing sensory stimuli
D. Applying ankle and wrist restraints

Correct Answer: A

Explanation/Reference:

(A) These clients are at high risk for seizures during the 1st week after cessation of alcohol intake. (B) Fluid intake should be increased to prevent dehydration. (C) Environmental stimuli should be decreased to prevent precipitation of seizures. (D) Application of restraints may cause the client to increase his or her physical activity and may eventually lead to exhaustion.

QUESTION 149

A psychotic client who believes that he is God and rules all the universe is experiencing which type of delusion?

A. Somatic
B. Grandiose

C. Persecutory

D. Nihilistic

Correct Answer: B

Explanation/Reference:

(A) These delusions are related to the belief that an individual has an incurable illness.
(B) These delusions are related to feelings of self-importance and uniqueness.
 (C) These delusions are related to feelings of being conspired against.
(D) These delusions are related to denial of self-existence.

QUESTION 150

A client confides to the nurse that he tasted poison in his evening meal. This would be an example of what type of hallucination?

A. Auditory

B. Gustatory

C. Olfactory

D. Visceral

Correct Answer: B

Explanation/Reference:

(A) Auditory hallucinations involve sensory perceptions of hearing.
(B) Gustatory hallucinations involve sensory perceptions of taste.
(C) Olfactory hallucinations involve sensory perceptions of smell.
 (D) Visceral hallucinations involve sensory perceptions of sensation.

QUESTION 151

A schizophrenic client has made sexual overtures toward her physician on numerous occasions.

During lunch, the client tells the nurse, "My doctor is in love with me and wants to marry me." This client is using which of the following defense mechanisms?

A. Displacement
B. Projection
C. Reaction formation
D. Suppression

Correct Answer: B

Explanation/Reference:

(A) Displacement involves transferring feelings to a more acceptable object.
(B) Projection involves attributing one's thoughts or feelings to another person.
(C) Reaction formation involves transforming an unacceptable impulse into the opposite behavior.
(D) Suppression involves the intentional exclusion of unpleasant thoughts or experiences.

QUESTION 152

Hypoxia is the primary problem related to near-drowning victims. The first organ that sustains irreversible damage after submersion in water is the:

A. Kidney (urinary system)
B. Brain (nervous system)
C. Heart (circulatory system)
D. Lungs (respiratory system)

Correct Answer: B

Explanation/Reference:

(A) The kidney can survive after 30 minutes of water submersion.
(B) The cerebral neurons sustain irreversible damage after 46 minutes of water submersion.
(C) The heart can survive up to 30 minutes of water submersion.
(D) The lungs can survive up to 30 minutes of water submersion.

QUESTION 153

One of the most dramatic and serious complications associated with bacterial meningitis is Waterhouse- Friderichsen syndrome, which is:

A. Peripheral circulatory collapse
B. Syndrome of inappropriate antiduretic hormone
C. Cerebral edema resulting in hydrocephalus
D. Auditory nerve damage resulting in permanent hearing loss

Correct Answer: A

Explanation/Reference:

(A) Waterhouse-Friderichsen syndrome is peripheral circulatory collapse, which may result in extensive and diffuse intravascular coagulation and thrombocytopenia resulting in death.
(B) Syndrome of inappropriate antidiuretic hormone is a complication of meningitis, but it is not Waterhouse- Friderichsen syndrome.
(C) Cerebral edema resulting in hydrocephalus is a complication of meningitis, but it is not Waterhouse-Friderichsen syndrome.
(D) Auditory nerve damage resulting in permanent hearing loss is a complication of meningitis, but it is not Waterhouse- Friderichsen syndrome.

QUESTION 154

An 8-year-old child comes to the physician's office complaining of swelling and pain in the knees. His mother says, "The swelling occurred for no reason, and it keeps getting worse." The initial diagnosis is Lyme disease. When talking to the mother and child, questions related to which of the following would be important to include in the initial history?

A. A decreased urinary output and flank pain
B. A fever of over 103F occurring over the last 23 weeks

C. Rashes covering the palms of the hands and the soles of the feet
D. Headaches, malaise, or sore throat

Correct Answer: D

Explanation/Reference:

(A) Urinary tract symptoms are not commonly associated with Lyme disease.
(B) A fever of 103F is not characteristic of Lyme disease.
(C) The rash that is associated with Lyme disease does not appear on the palms of the hands and the soles of the feet.
(D) Classic symptoms of Lyme disease include headache, malaise, fatigue, anorexia, stiff neck, generalized lymphadenopathy, splenomegaly, conjunctivitis, sore throat, abdominal pain, and cough.

QUESTION 155

The most commonly known vectors of Lyme disease are:

A. Mites
B. Fleas
C. Ticks
D. Mosquitoes

Correct Answer: C

Explanation/Reference:

(A) Mites are not the common vector of Lyme disease.
(B) Fleas are not the common vector of Lyme disease.
(C) Ticks are the common vector of Lyme disease.
(D) Mosquitoes are not the common vector of Lyme disease.

QUESTION 156

A laboratory technique specific for diagnosing Lyme disease is:

A. Polymerase chain reaction
B. Heterophil antibody test
C. Decreased serum calcium level
D. Increased serum potassium level

Correct Answer: A

Explanation/Reference:

(A) Polymerase chain reaction is the laboratory technique specific for Lyme disease.
(B) Heterophil antibody test is used to diagnose mononucleosis.
(C) Lyme disease does not decrease the serum calcium level.
(D) Lyme disease does not increase the serum potassium level.

QUESTION 157

The nurse would expect to include which of the following when planning the management of the client with Lyme disease?

A. Complete bed rest for 68 weeks
B. Tetracycline treatment
C. IV amphotericin B
D. High-protein diet with limited fluids

Correct Answer: B

Explanation/Reference:

(A) The client is not placed on complete bed rest for 6 weeks.
(B) Tetracycline is the treatment of choice for children with Lyme disease who are over the age of 9.
(C) IV amphotericin B is the treatment for histoplasmosis.
(D) The client is not restricted to a high-protein diet with limited fluids.

QUESTION 158

A 3-year-old child is hospitalized with burns covering her trunk and lower extremities. Which of the following would the nurse use to assess adequacy of fluid resuscitation in the burned child?

A. Blood pressure
B. Serum potassium level
C. Urine output
D. Pulse rate

Correct Answer: C

Explanation/Reference:

(A) Blood pressure can remain normotensive even in a state of hypovolemia.
(B) Serum potassium is not reliable for determining adequacy of fluid resuscitation.
(C) Urine output, alteration in sensorium, and capillary refill are the most reliable indicators for assessing adequacy of fluid resuscitation.
(D) Pulse rate may vary for many reasons and is not a reliable indicator for assessing adequacy of fluid resuscitation.

QUESTION 159

Proper positioning for the child who is in Bryant's traction is:

A. Both hips flexed at a 90-degree angle with the knees extended and the buttocks elevated off the bed
B. Both legs extended, and the hips are not flexed
C. The affected leg extended with slight hip flexion
D. Both hips and knees maintained at a 90-degree flexion angle, and the back flat on the bed

Correct Answer: A

Explanation/Reference:

(A) The child's weight supplies the counter traction for Bryant's traction; the buttocks are slightly elevated off the bed, and the hips are flexed at a 90-degree angle. Both legs are suspended by skin traction.

(B) The child in Buck's extension traction maintains the legs extended and parallel to the bed.

(C) The child in Russell traction maintains hip flexion of the affected leg at the prescribed angle with the leg extended.

(D) The child in "9090" traction maintains both hips and knees at a 90-degree flexion angle and the back is flat on the bed.

QUESTION 160

A child sustains a supracondylar fracture of the femur. When assessing for vascular injury, the nurse should be alert for the signs of ischemia, which include:

A. Bleeding, bruising, and hemorrhage
B. Increase in serum levels of creatinine, alkaline phosphatase, and aspartate transaminase
C. Pain, pallor, pulselessness, paresthesia, and paralysis
D. Generalized swelling, pain, and diminished functional use with muscle rigidityand crepitus

Correct Answer: C

Explanation/Reference:

(A) Bleeding, bruising, and hemorrhage may occur due to injury but are not classic signs of ischemia.
(B) An increase in serum levels of creatinine, alkaline phosphatase, and aspartate transaminase is related to the disruption of muscle integrity.
(C) Classic signs of ischemia related to vascular injury secondary to long bone fractures include the five "P's": pain, pallor, pulselessness, paresthesia, and paralysis.
(D) Generalized swelling, pain, and diminished functional use with muscle rigidity and crepitus are common clinical manifestations of a fracture but not ischemia.

QUESTION 161

When administering phenytoin (Dilantin) to a child, the nurse should be aware that a toxic effect of phenytoin therapy is:

A. Stephens-Johnson syndrome

B. Folate deficiency
C. Leukopenic aplastic anemia
D. Granulocytosis and nephrosis

Correct Answer: A

Explanation/Reference:

(A) Stephens-Johnson syndrome is a toxic effect of phenytoin.
(B) Folate deficiency is a side effect of phenytoin, but not a toxic effect.
(C) Leukopenic aplastic anemia is a toxic effect of carbamazepine (Tegretol).
(D) Granulocytosis and nephrosis are toxic effects of trimethadione (Tridione).

QUESTION 162

A six-month-old infant has been admitted to the emergency room with febrile seizures. In the teaching of the parents, the nurse states that:

A. Sustained temperature elevation over 103F is generally related to febrile seizures
B. Febrile seizures do not usually recur
C. There is little risk of neurological deficit and mental retardation as sequelae to febrile seizures
D. Febrile seizures are associated with diseases of the central nervous system

Correct Answer: C

Explanation/Reference:

(A) The temperature elevation related to febrile seizures generally exceeds 101F, and seizures occur during the temperature rise rather than after a prolonged elevation.
(B) Febrile seizures may recur and are more likely to do so when the first seizure occurs in the 1st year of life.
(C)There is little risk of neurological deficit, mental retardation, or

altered behavior secondary to febrile seizures.
(D) Febrile seizures are associated with disease of the central nervous system.

QUESTION 163

When assessing a child with diabetes insipidus, the nurse should be aware of the cardinal signs of:

A. Anemia and vomiting
B. Polyuria and polydipsia
C. Irritability relieved by feeding formula
D. Hypothermia and azotemia

Correct Answer: B

Explanation/Reference:

(A) Anemia and vomiting are not cardinal signs of diabetes insipidus.
(B) Polyuria and polydipsia are the cardinal signs of diabetes insipidus.
(C) Irritability relieved by feeding water, not formula, is a common sign, but not the cardinal sign, of diabetes insipidus.
(D) Hypothermia and azotemia are signs, but not cardinal signs, of diabetes insipidus.

QUESTION 164

The usual treatment for diabetes insipidus is with IM or SC injection of vasopressin tannate in oil. Nursing care related to the client receiving IM vasopressin tannate would include:

A. Weigh once a week and report to the physician any weight gain of 10 lb.
B. Limit fluid intake to 500 mL/day.
C. Store the medication in a refrigerator and allow to stand at room temperature for 30 minutes prior to administration.
D. Hold the vial under warm water for 1015 minutes and shake vigorously before drawing medication into the syringe.

Correct Answer: D

Explanation/Reference:

(A) Weight should be obtained daily.
(B) Fluid is not restricted but is given according to urine output.
(C) The medication does not have to be stored in a refrigerator.
(D) Holding the vial under warm water for 1015 minutes or rolling between your hands and shaking vigorously before drawing medication into the syringe activates the medication in the oil solution.

QUESTION 165

A child is admitted to the emergency room with her mother. Her mother states that she has been exposed to chickenpox. During the assessment, the nurse would note a characteristic rash:

A. That is covered with vesicular scabs all in the macular stage
B. That appears profusely on the trunk and sparsely on the extremities
C. That first appears on the neck and spreads downward
D. That appears especially on the cheeks, which gives a"slapped-cheek" appearance

Correct Answer: B

Explanation/Reference:

(A) A rash with vesicular scabs in all stages (macule, papule, vesicle, and crusts).
(B) A rash that appears profusely on the trunk and sparsely on the extremities.

(C) A rash that first appears on the neck and spreads downward is characteristic of rubeola and rubella.
(D) A rash, especially on the cheeks, that gives a "slapped-cheek" appearance is characteristic of roseola.

QUESTION 166

Discharge teaching was effective if the parents of a child with atopic dermatitis could state the importance of:

A. Maintaining a high-humidified environment
B. Furry, soft stuffed animals for play
C. Showering 34 times a day
D. Wrapping hands in soft cotton gloves

Correct Answer: D

Explanation/Reference:

(A) Maintaining a low-humidified environment.
(B) Avoiding furry, soft stuffed animals for play, which may increase symptoms of allergy.
(C) Avoiding showering, which irritates the dermatitis, and encouraging bathing 4 times a day in colloid bath for temporary relief
(D) Wrapping hands in soft cotton gloves to prevent skin damage during scratching.

QUESTION 167

The priority nursing goal when working with an autistic child is:

A. To establish trust with the child
B. To maintain communication with the family
C. To promote involvement in school activities
D. To maintain nutritional requirements

Correct Answer: A

Explanation/Reference:

(A) The priority nursing goal when working with an autistic child is establishing a trusting relationship.
(B) Maintaining a relationship with the family is important but having the trust of the child is a priority.

(C) To promote involvement in school activities is inappropriate for a child who is autistic.
(D) Maintaining nutritional requirements is not the primary problem of the autistic child.

QUESTION 168

The child with iron poisoning is given IV deforoxamine mesylate (Desferal). Following administration, the child suffers hypotension, facial flushing, and urticaria. The initial nursing intervention would be to:

A. Discontinue the IV
B. Stop the medication, and begin a normal saline infusion
C. Take all vital signs, and report to the physician
D. Assess urinary output, and if it is 30 mL an hour, maintain current treatment

Correct Answer: B

Explanation/Reference:

(A) The IV line should not be discontinued because other IV medications will be needed.
(B) Stop the medication and begin a normal saline infusion. The child is exhibiting signs of an allergic reaction and could go into shock if the medication is not stopped. The line should be kept opened for other medication.
(C) Taking vital signs and reporting to the physician is not an adequate intervention because the IV medication continues to flow.
(D) Assessing urinary output and, if it is 30 mL an hour, maintaining current treatment is an inappropriate intervention owing to the child's obvious allergic reaction.

QUESTION 169

As the nurse assesses a male adolescent with chlamydia, the nurse determines that a sign of chlamydia is:

A. Enlarged penis
B. Secondary lymphadenitis
C. Epididymitis
D. Hepatomegaly

Correct Answer: C

Explanation/Reference:

(A) An enlarged penis is not a sign of chlamydia.
(B) Secondary lymphadenitis is a complication of lymphogranuloma venereum.
(C) Untreated chlamydial infection can spread from the urethra, causing epididymitis, which presents as a tender, scrotal swelling.

(D) Hepatomegaly is not a complication.

QUESTION 170

When teaching a mother of a 4-month-old with diarrhea about the importance of preventing dehydration, the nurse would inform the mother about the importance of feeding her child:

A. Fruit juices
B. Diluted carbonated drinks
C. Soy-based, lactose-free formula
D. Regular formulas mixed with electrolyte solutions

Correct Answer: C

Explanation/Reference:

(A) Diluted fruit juices are not recommended for rehydration because they tend to aggravate the diarrhea.
(B) Diluted soft drinks have a high-carbohydrate content, which aggravates the diarrhea.
(C) Soy-based, lactose-free formula reduces stool output and duration of diarrhea in most infants.
(D) Regular formulas contain lactose, which can increase diarrhea.

QUESTION 171

The primary reason that an increase in heart rate (100 bpm) detrimental to the client with a myocardial infarction (MI) is that:

A. Stroke volume and blood pressure will drop proportionately
B. Systolic ejection time will decrease, thereby decreasing cardiac output
C. Decreased contractile strength will occur due to decreased filling time
D. Decreased coronary artery perfusion due to decreased diastolic filling time will occur, which will increase ischemic damage to the myocardium

Correct Answer: D
Explanation/Reference:

(A) Decreased stroke volume and blood pressure will occur secondary to decreased diastolic filling.
(B) Tachycardia primarily decreases diastole; systolic time changes very little.
(C) Contractility decreases owing to the decreased filling time and decreased time for fiber lengthening.
(D) Decreased O2 supply due to decreased time for filling of the coronary arteries increases ischemia and infarct size. Tachycardia primarily robs the heart of diastolic time, which is the primary time for coronary artery filling.

QUESTION 172

To appropriately monitor therapy and client progress, the nurse should be aware that increased myocardial work and O2 demand will occur with which of the following?

A. Positive inotropic therapy
B. Negative chronotropic therapy
C. Increase in balance of myocardial O2 supply and demand
D. Afterload reduction therapy

Correct Answer: A

Explanation/Reference:

(A) Inotropic therapy will increase contractility, which will increase myocardial O2 demand.
(B) Decreased heart rate to the point of bradycardia will increase coronary artery filling time. Thisshould be used cautiously because tachycardia may be a compensatory mechanism to increase cardiac output.
(C) The goal in the care of the MI client with angina is to maintain a balance between myocardial O2 supply and demand.
(D)Decrease in systemic vascular resistance by drug therapy, such as IV nitroglycerin or nitroprusside, or intra-aortic balloon pump therapy, would decrease myocardial work and O2 demand.

QUESTION 173

The nurse would need to monitor the serum glucose levels of a client receiving which of the following medications, owing to its effects on glycogenolysis and insulin release?

A. Norepinephrine (Levophed)
B. Dobutamine (Dobutrex)
C. Propranolol (Inderal)
D. Epinephrine (Adrenalin)

Correct Answer: D

Explanation/Reference:

(A) Norepinephrine's side effects are primarily related to safe, effective care environment and include decreased peripheral perfusion and bradycardia.
(B) Dobutamine's side effects include increased heart rate and blood pressure, ventricular ectopy, nausea, and headache.
(C) Propranolol's side effects include elevated blood urea nitrogen, serum transaminase, alkaline phosphatase, and lactic dehydrogenase.
(D)Epinephrine increases serum glucose levels by increasing glycogenolysis and inhibiting insulin release. Prolonged use can elevate serum lactate levels, leading to metabolic acidosis, increased urinary catecholamines, false elevation of blood urea nitrogen, and decreased coagulation time.

QUESTION 174

Which of the following medications requires close observation for bronchospasm in the client with chronic obstructive pulmonary disease or asthma?

A. Verapamil (Isoptin)
B. Amrinone (Inocor)
C. Epinephrine (Adrenalin)
D. Propranolol (Inderal)

Correct Answer: D

Explanation/Reference:

(A) Verapamil has the respiratory side effect of nasal or chest congestion, dyspnea, shortness of breath (SOB), and wheezing.
(B) Amrinone has the effect of increased contractility and dilation of the vascular smooth muscle. It has no noted respiratory side effects.
(C) Epinephrine has the effect of bronchodilation through stimulation.
(D) Propranolol, esmolol, and labetalol are all - blocking agents, which can increase airway resistance and cause bronchospasms.

QUESTION 175

The following medications were noted on review of the client's home medication profile. Which of the medications would most likely potentiate or elevate serum digoxin levels?

A. KCl
B. Thyroid agents
C. Quinidine
D. Theophylline

Correct Answer: C

Explanation/Reference:

(A) Hypokalemia can cause digoxin toxicity. Administration of KCl would prevent this.
(B) Thyroid agents decrease digoxin levels.
(C) Quinidine increases digoxin levels dramatically.
(D) Theophylline is not noted to have an effect on digoxin levels.

QUESTION 176

In the client with a diagnosis of coronary artery disease, the nurse would anticipate the complication of bradycardia with occlusion of which coronary artery?

A. Right coronary artery
B. Left main coronary artery
C. Circumflex coronary artery
D. Left anterior descending coronary artery

Correct Answer: A
Explanation/Reference:

(A) Sinus bradycardia and atrioventricular (AV) heart block are usually a result of right coronary artery occlusion. The right coronary artery perfuses the sinoatrial and AV nodes in most individuals.

(B) Occlusion of the left main coronary artery causes bundle branch blocks and premature ventricular contractions.

(C) Occlusion of the circumflex artery does not cause bradycardia.

(D) Sinus tachycardia occurs primarily with left anterior descending coronary artery occlusion because this form of occlusion impairs left ventricular function.

QUESTION 177

When inspecting a cardiovascular client, the nurse notes that he needs to sit upright to breathe. This behavior is most indicative of:

A. Pericarditis
B. Anxiety
C. Congestive heart failure
D. Angina

Correct Answer: C

Explanation/Reference:

(A) Pericarditis can cause dyspnea but primarily causes chest pain. (B) Anxiety can cause dyspnea resulting in SOB, yet it is not typically influenced by degree of head elevation. (C) The inability to oxygenate well without being upright is most indicative of congestive heart failure, due to alveolar drowning. (D) Angina causes primarily chest pain; any

SOB associated with angina is not influenced by body position.

QUESTION 178

When a client questions the nurse as to the purpose of exercise electrocardiography (ECG) in the diagnosis of cardiovascular disorders, the nurse's response should be based on the fact that:

A. The test provides a baseline for further tests
B. The procedure simulates usual daily activity and myocardial performance
C. The client can be monitored while cardiac conditioning and heart toning are done
D. Ischemia can be diagnosed because exercise increasesO2 consumption and demand

Correct Answer: D

Explanation/Reference:

(A) The purpose of the study is not to provide a baseline for further tests.
(B) The test causes an increase in O2 demand beyond that required to perform usual daily activities.
(C) Monitoring does occur, but the test is not for the purpose of cardiac toning and conditioning.
(D) Exercise ECG, or stress testing, is designed to elevate the peripheral and myocardial needs for O2 to evaluate the ability of the myocardium and coronary arteries to meet the additional demands.

QUESTION 179

In assessing cardiovascular clients with progression of aortic stenosis, the nurse should be aware that there is typically:

A. Decreased pulmonary blood flow and cyanosis
B. Increased pressure in the pulmonary veins and pulmonary edema
C. Systemic venous engorgement
D. Increased left ventricular systolic pressures and hypertrophy

Correct Answer: D

Explanation/Reference:

(A) These signs are seen in pulmonic stenosis or in response to pulmonary congestion and edema and mitral stenosis.
(B) These signs are seen primarily in mitral stenosis or as a late sign in aortic stenosis after left ventricular failure.
(C) These signs are seen primarily in right-sided heart valve dysfunction.
(D) Left ventricular hypertrophy occurs to increase muscle mass and overcome the stenosis; left ventricular pressures increase as left ventricular volume increases owing to insufficient emptying.

QUESTION 180

The cardiac client who exhibits the symptoms of disorientation, lethargy, and seizures may be exhibiting a toxic reaction to:

A. Digoxin (Lanoxin)
B. Lidocaine (Xylocaine)
C. Quinidine gluconate or sulfate (Quinaglute, Quinidex)
D. Nitroglycerin IV (Tridil)

Correct Answer: B

Explanation/Reference:

(A) Side effects of digoxin include headache, hypotension, AV block, blurred vision, and yellow-green halos.
(B) Side effects of lidocaine include heart block, headache, dizziness, confusion, tremor, lethargy, and convulsions.
(C) Side effects of quinidine include heart block, hepatotoxicity, thrombocytopenia, and respiratory depression.
(D) Side effects of nitroglycerin include postural hypotension, headache, dizziness, and flushing.

QUESTION 181

Which of the following ECG changes would be seen as a positive myocardial stress test response?

A. Hyperacute T wave
B. Prolongation of the PR interval
C. ST-segment depression
D. Pathological Q wave

Correct Answer: C

Explanation/Reference:

(A) Hyperacute T waves occur with hyperkalemia.
(B) Prolongation of the P R interval occurs with first- degree AV block.
(C) Horizontal ST-segment depression of>1 mm during exercise is definitely a positive criterion on the exercise ECG test.
 (D) Patho-logical Q waves occur with MI.

QUESTION 182

Assessment of the client with pericarditis may reveal which of the following?

A. Ventricular gallop and substernal chest pain
B. Narrowed pulse pressure and shortness of breath
C. Pericardial friction rub and pain on deep inspiration
D. Pericardial tamponade and widened pulse pressure

Correct Answer: C

Explanation/Reference:

(A) No S3 or S4 are noted with pericarditis.
(B) No change in pulse pressure occurs.
(C) The symptoms of pericarditis vary with the cause, but they usually include chest pain, dyspnea, tachycardia, rise in temperature, and friction rub caused by fibrin or other deposits. The pain seen with pericarditis typically worsens with deep inspiration.
(D) Tamponade is not typically seen early on, and no change in pulse pressure occurs.

QUESTION 183

Clinical manifestations seen in left-sided rather than in right-sided heart failure are:

A. Elevated central venous pressure and peripheral edema
B. Dyspnea and jaundice
C. Hypotension and hepatomegaly
D. Decreased peripheral perfusion and rales

Correct Answer: D

Explanation/Reference:

(A, B, C) Clinical manifestations of right-sided heart failure are weakness, peripheral edema, jugular venous distention, hepatomegaly, jaundice, and elevated central venous pressure.
(D) Clinical manifestations of left-sided heart failure are left ventricular dysfunction, decreased cardiac output, hypotension, and the backward failure as a result of increased left atrium and pulmonary artery pressures, pulmonary edema, and rales.

QUESTION 184

Which classification of drugs is contraindicated for the client with hypertrophic cardiomyopathy?

A. Positive inotropes
B. Vasodilators
C. Diuretics
D. Antidysrhythmics

Correct Answer: A

Explanation/Reference:

(A) Positive inotropic agents should not be administered owing to their action of increasing myocardial contractility. Increased ventricular contractility would increase outflow tract obstruction in the client with hypertrophic cardiomyopathy.
(B) Vasodilators are not typically prescribed but are not contraindicated.

(C) Diuretics are used with caution to avoid causing hypovolemia.
(D) Antidysrhythmics are typically needed to treat both atrial and
ventricular dysrhythmias.

QUESTION 185

To ensure proper client education, the nurse should teach the client
taking SL nitroglycerin to expect which of the following responses with
administration?

A. Stinging, burning when placed under the tongue
B. Temporary blurring of vision
C. Generalized urticaria with prolonged use
D. Urinary frequency

Correct Answer: A

Explanation/Reference:

(A) Stinging or burning when nitroglycerin is placed under the tongue is
to be expected. This effect indicates that the medication is potent and
effective for use. Failure to have this response means that the client
needs to get a new bottle of nitroglycerin.
(B, C, D) The other responses are not expected in this situation and
are not even side effects.

QUESTION 186

When a client is receiving vasoactive therapy IV, such as dopamine
(Intropin), and extravasation occurs, the nurse should be prepared to
administer which of the following medications directly into the site?

A. Phentolamine (Regitine)
B. Epinephrine
C. Phenylephrine (Neo-Synephrine)
D. Sodium bicarbonate

Correct Answer: A

Explanation/Reference:

(A) Phentolamine is given to counteract the -adrenergic effects that cause ischemia and necrosis of local tissue.
 (B) Epinephrine is an endogenous catecholamine that produces vasoconstriction and increases heart rate and contractility.
(C) Phenylephrine causes constriction of arterioles of skin, mucous membranes, and viscera, which in turn can cause ischemia and necrosis.
(D) Sodium bicarbonate is an alkalinizing agent that is incompatible with dopamine.

QUESTION 187

Which of the following would differentiate acute from chronic respiratory acidosis in the assessment of the trauma client?

A. Increased PaCO2
B. Decreased PaO2
C. Increased HCO3
D. Decreased base excess

Correct Answer: C

Explanation/Reference:

(A) Increased CO2 will occur in both acute and chronic respiratory acidosis.
(B) Hypoxia does not determine acid-base status.
(C) Elevation of HCO3 is a compensatory mechanism in acidosis that occurs almost immediately, but it takes hours to show any effect and days to reach maximum compensation. Renal disease and diuretic therapy may impair the ability of the kidneys to compensate.
(D) Base excess is a nonrespiratory contributor to acid-base balance. It would increase to compensate for acidosis.

QUESTION 188

Which of the following signs and symptoms indicates a tension pneumothorax as compared to an open pneumothorax?

A. Ventilation-perfusion (V./Q.) mismatch
B. Hypoxemia and respiratory acidosis

C. Mediastinal tissue and organ shifting
D. Decreased tidal volume and tachypnea

Correct Answer: C

Explanation/Reference:

(A, B, D) These occur in both tension pneumothorax and open
pneumothorax.
(C) The tension pneumothorax acts like a one- way valve so that the
pneumothorax increases with each breath. Eventually, it occupies
enough space to shift mediastinal tissue toward the unaffected side
away from the midline.
Tracheal deviation, movement of point of maximum impulse, and
decreased cardiac output will occur. The other three options will occur
in both types of pneumothorax.

QUESTION 189

Hematotympanum and otorrhea are associated with which of the
following head injuries?

A. Basilar skull fracture
B. Subdural hematoma
C. Epidural hematoma
D. Frontal lobe fracture

Correct Answer: A

Explanation/Reference:

(A) Basilar skull fractures are fractures of the base of the skull. Blood
behind the eardrum or blood or cerebrospinal fluid (CSF) leaking from
the ear are indicative of a dural laceration. Basilar skull fractures are
the only type with these symptoms.
(B, C, D) These do not typically cause dural lacerations and CSF
leakage.

QUESTION 190

A client with a C-34 fracture has just arrived in the emergency room. The primary nursing intervention is:

A. Stabilization of the cervical spine
B. Airway assessment and stabilization
C. Confirmation of spinal cord injury
D. Normalization of intravascular volume

Correct Answer: B

Explanation/Reference:

(A) If cervical spine injury is suspected, the airway should be maintained using the jaw thrust method that also protects the cervical spine.
(B) Primary intervention is protection of the airway and adequate ventilation.
(C, D) All other interventions are secondary to adequate ventilation.

QUESTION 191

In a client with chest trauma, the nurse needs to evaluate mediastinal position. This can best be done by:
A. Auscultating bilateral breath sounds
B. Palpating for presence of crepitus
C. Palpating for trachial deviation
D. Auscultating heart sounds

Correct Answer: C

Explanation/Reference:

(A) No change in the breath sounds occurs as a direct result of the mediastinal shift.
(B) Crepitus can occur owing to the primary disorder, not to the mediastinal shift.

(C) Mediastinal shift occurs primarily with tension pneumothorax, but it can occur with very large hemothorax or pneumothorax. Mediastinal shift causes trachial deviation and deviation of the heart's point of maximum impulse.
(D) No change in the heart sounds occurs as a result of the mediastinal shift.

QUESTION 192

Priapism may be a sign of:

A. Altered neurological function
B. Imminent death
C. Urinary incontinence
D. Reproductive dysfunction

Correct Answer: A

Explanation/Reference:

(A) Priapism in the trauma client is due to the neurological dysfunction seen in spinal cord injury. Priapism is an abnormal erection of the penis; it may be accompanied by pain and tenderness. This may disappear as spinal cord edema is relieved.
(B) Priapism is not associated with death.
(C) Urinary retention, rather than incontinence, may occur.
(D) Reproductive dysfunction may be a secondary problem.

QUESTION 193

When evaluating a client with symptoms of shock, it is important for the nurse to differentiate between neurogenic and hypovolemic shock. The symptoms of neurogenic shock differ from hypovolemic shock in that:

A. In neurogenic shock, the skin is warm and dry
B. In hypovolemic shock, there is a bradycardia
C. In hypovolemic shock, capillary refill is less than 2 seconds
D. In neurogenic shock, there is delayed capillary refill

Correct Answer: A

(A) Neurogenic shock is caused by injury to the cervical region, which leads to loss of sympathetic control. This loss leads to vasodilation of the vascular beds, bradycardia resulting from the lack of sympathetic balance to parasympathetic stimuli from the vagus nerve, and the loss of the ability to sweat below the level of injury. In neurogenic shock, the client is hypotensive but bradycardiac with warm, dry skin.
(B) In hypovolemic shock, the client is hypotensive and tachycardiac with cool skin.
(C) In hypovolemic shock, the capillary refill would be>5 seconds.
(D) In neurogenic shock, there is no capillary delay, the vascular beds are dilated, and peripheral flow is good.

QUESTION 194

Which of the following would have the physiological effect of decreasing intracranial pressure (ICP)?

A. Increased core body temperature
B. Decreased serum osmolality
C. Administration of hypo-osmolar fluids
D. Decreased PaCO2

Correct Answer: D

Explanation/Reference:

(A) An increase in core body temperature increases metabolism and results in an increase in ICP.
(B) Decreased serum osmolality indicates a fluid overload and may result in an increase in ICP.
(C) Hypo- osmolar fluids are generally voided in the neurologically compromised. Using IV fluids such as D5W results in the dextrose being metabolized, releasing free water that is absorbed by the brain cells, leading to cerebral edema.
(D) Hypercapnia and hypoventilation, which cause retention of CO2 and lead to respiratory acidosis, both increase ICP. CO2 is the most potent vasodilator known.

QUESTION 195

A client who has sustained a basilar skull fracture exhibits blood-tinged
drainage from his nose. After establishing a clear airway, administering
supplemental O2, and establishing IV access, the next nursing
intervention would be to:

A. Pass a nasogastric tube through the left nostril
B. Place a 4 X 4 gauze in the nares to impede the flow
C. Gently suction the nasal drainage to protect the airway
D. Perform a halo test and glucose level on the drainage

Correct Answer: D

Explanation/Reference:

(A) Basilar skull fracture may cause dural lacerations, which result in
CSF leaking from the ears or nose. Insertion of a tube could lead to
CSF going into the brain tissue or sinuses.
(B) Tamponading flow could worsen the problem and increase ICP.
(C) Suction could increase brain damage and dislocate tissue.
 (D) Testing the fluid from the nares would determine the presence of
CSF. Elevation of the head, notification of the medical staff, and
prophylactic antibiotics are appropriate therapy.

QUESTION 196

A client with a diagnosis of C-4 injury has been stabilized and is ready
for discharge. Because this client is at risk for autonomic dysreflexia,
he and his family should be instructed to assess for and report:

A. Dizziness and tachypnea
B. Circumoral pallor and lightheadedness
C. Headache and facial flushing
D. Pallor and itching of the face and neck

Correct Answer: C

Explanation/Reference:

(A) Tachypnea is not a symptom.
(B) Circumoral pallor is not a symptom.
(C) Autonomic dysreflexia is an uninhibited and exaggerated reflex of the autonomic nervous system to stimulation, which results in vasoconstriction and elevated blood pressure.
(D) Pallor and itching are not symptoms.

QUESTION 197

The initial treatment for a client with a liquid chemical burn injury is to:

A. Irrigate the area with neutralizing solutions
B. Flush the exposed area with large amounts of water
C. Inject calcium chloride into the burned area
D. Apply lanolin ointment to the area

Correct Answer: B

Explanation/Reference:

(A) In the past, neutralizing solutions were recommended, but presently there is concern that these solutions extend the depth of burn area.
(B) The use of large amounts of water to flush the area is recommended for chemical burns.
(C) Calcium chloride is not recommended therapy and would likely worsen the problem.
 (D) Lanolin is of no benefit in the initial treatment of a chemical injury and may actually extend a thermal injury.

QUESTION 198

The most important reason to closely assess circumferential burns at least every hour is that they may result in:

A. Hypovolemia
B. Renal damage
C. Ventricular arrhythmias
D. Loss of peripheral pulses

Correct Answer: D

Explanation/Reference:

(A) Hypovolemia could be a result of fluid loss from thermal injury, but not as a result of the circumferential injury.
(B) Renal damage is typically seen because of prolonged hypovolemia or myoglobinuria.
(C) Electrical injuries and electrolyte changes typically cause arrhythmias in the burn client.

(D) Full-thickness circumferential burns are nonelastic and result in an internal tourniquet effect that compromises distal blood flow when the area involved is an extremity. Circumferential full- thickness torso burns compromise respiratory motion and, when extreme, cardiac return.

QUESTION 199

During burn therapy, morphine is primarily administered IV for pain management because this route:

A. Delays absorption to provide continuous pain relief
B. Facilitates absorption because absorption from muscles is not dependable
C. Allows for discontinuance of the medication if respiratory depression develops
D. Avoids causing additional pain from IM injections

Correct Answer: B

Explanation/Reference:

(A) Absorption would be increased, not decreased.
(B) IM injections should not be used until the client is hemodynamically stable and has adequate tissue perfusion. Medications will remain in the subcutaneous tissue with the fluid that is present in the interstitial spaces in the acute phase of the thermal injury. The client will have a poor response to the medication administered, and a "dumping" of the medication can occur when the medication and fluid are shifted back into the intravascular spaces in the next phase of healing.
(C) IV administration of the medication would hasten respiratory compromise, if present.
(D) The desire to avoid causing the client additional pain is not a primary reason for this route of administration.

QUESTION 200

The medication that best penetrates eschar is:

A. Mafenide acetate (Sulfamylon)
B. Silver sulfadiazine(Silvadene)
C. Neomycin sulfate(Neosporin)
D. Povidone-iodine (Betadine)

Correct Answer: A

Explanation/Reference:

(A) Mafenide acetate is bacteriostatic against gram-positive and gram-negative organisms and is the agent that best penetrates eschar.
(B) Silver sulfadiazine poorly penetrates eschar.
(C) Neomycin sulfate does not penetrate eschar.
(D) Povidoneiodine does not penetrate eschar.

QUESTION 201

When the nurse is evaluating lab data for a client 1824 hours after a major thermal burn, the expected physiological changes would include which of the following?

A. Elevated serum sodium
B. Elevated serum calcium
C. Elevated serum protein
D. Elevated hematocrit

Correct Answer: D

Explanation/Reference:

(A) Sodium enters the edema fluid in the burned area, lowering the sodium content of the vascular fluid. Hyponatremia may continue for days to several weeks because of sodium loss to edema, sodium shifting into the cells, and later, diuresis.
(B) Hypocalcemia occurs because of calcium loss to edema fluid at the burned site (third space fluid).

(C) Protein loss occurs at the burn site owing to increased capillary permeability. Serum protein levels remain low until healing occurs.
(D) Hematocrit level is elevated owing to hemoconcentration from hypovolemia. Anemia is present in the postburn stage owing to blood loss and hemolysis, but it cannot be assessed until the client is adequately hydrated.

QUESTION 202

The nurse notes hyperventilation in a client with a thermal injury. She recognizes that this may be a reaction to which of the following medications if applied in large amounts?

A. Neosporin sulfate
B. Mafenide acetate
C. Silver sulfadiazine
D. Povidone-iodine

Correct Answer: B

Explanation/Reference:

(A) The side effects of neomycin sulfate include rash, urticaria, nephrotoxicity, and ototoxicity.
(B) The side effects of mafenide acetate include bone marrow suppression, hemolytic anemia, eosinophilia, and metabolic acidosis. The hyperventilation is a compensatory response to the metabolic acidosis.
(C) The side effects of silver sulfadiazine include rash, itching, leukopenia, and decreased renal function.
(D) The primary side effect of povidone- iodine is decreased renal function.

QUESTION 203

The primary reason for sending a burn client home with a pressure garment, such as a Jobst garment, is that the garment:

A. Decreases hypertrophic scar formation
B. Assists with ambulation

C. Covers burn scars and decreases the psychological impact during recovery
D. Increases venous return and cardiac output by normalizing fluid status

Correct Answer: A

Explanation/Reference:

(A) Tubular support, such as that received with a Jobst garment, applies tension of 1020 mm Hg. This amount of uniform pressure is necessary to prevent or reduce hypertrophic scarring. Clients typically wear a pressure garment for 612 months during the recovery phase of their care.
(B) Pressure garments have no ambulatory assistive properties.
(C) Pressure garments can worsen the psychological impact of burn injury, especially if worn on the face.
(D) Pressure garments do not normalize fluid status.

QUESTION 204

A client with emphysema is placed on diuretics. In order to avoid potassium depletion as a side effect of the drug therapy, which of the following foods should be included in his diet?

A. Celery
B. Potatoes
C. Tomatoes
D. Liver

Correct Answer: B

Explanation/Reference:

(A) Celery is high in sodium.
(B) Potatoes are high in potassium.
(C) Tomatoes are high in sodium.
(D) Liver is high in iron.

QUESTION 205

Which of the following would the nurse expect to find following respiratory assessment of a client with advanced emphysema?

A. Distant breath sounds
B. Increased heart sounds
C. Decreased anteroposterior chest diameter
D. Collapsed neck veins

Correct Answer: A

Explanation/Reference:

(A) Distant breath sounds are found in clients with emphysema owing to increased anteroposterior chest diameter, overdistention, and air trapping.
(B) Deceased heart sounds are present because of the increased anteroposterior chest diameter.
(C) A barrel- shaped chest is characteristic of emphysema.
(D) Increased distention of neck veins is found owing to right-sided heart failure, which may be present in advanced emphysema.

QUESTION 206

The nurse assists a client with advanced emphysema to the bathroom. The client becomes extremely short of breath while returning to bed. The nurse should:

A. Increase his nasal O2 to 6 L/min
B. Place him in a lateral Sims' position
C. Encourage pursed-lip breathing
D. Have him breathe into a paper bag

Correct Answer: C

Explanation/Reference:

(A) Giving too high a concentration of O2 to a client with em-physema may remove his stimulus to breathe.
(B) The client should sit forward with his hands on his knees or an overbed table and with shoulders elevated.

(C) Pursed-lip breathing helps the client to blow off CO2 and to keep air passages open.
(D) Covering the face of a client extremely short of breath may cause anxiety and further increase dyspnea.

QUESTION 207

Signs and symptoms of an allergy attack include which of the following?

A. Wheezing on inspiration
B. Increased respiratory rate
C. Circumoral cyanosis
D. Prolonged expiration

Correct Answer: D

Explanation/Reference:

(A) Wheezing occurs during expiration when air movement is impaired because of constricted edematous bronchial lumina.
(B) Respirations are difficult, but the rate is frequently normal.
(C) The circumoral area is usually pale. Cyanosis is not an early sign of hypoxia.
(D) Expiration is prolonged because the alveoli are greatly distended and air trapping occurs.

QUESTION 208

A 55-year-old man is admitted to the hospital with complaints of fatigue, jaundice, anorexia, and clay- colored stools. His admitting diagnosis is "rule out hepatitis." Laboratory studies reveal elevated liver

enzymes and bilirubin. In obtaining his health history, the nurse should assess his potential for exposure to hepatitis.
Which of the following represents a high-risk group for contracting this disease?

A. Heterosexual males
B. Oncology nurses
C. American Indians
D. Jehovah's Witnesses

Correct Answer: B

Explanation/Reference:

(A) Homosexual males, not heterosexual males, are at high risk for
contracting hepatitis.
(B) Oncology nurses are employed in high-risk areas and perform
invasive procedures that expose them to potential sources of infection.
(C) The literature does not support the idea that any ethnic groups are
at higher risk.
(D) There is no evidence that any religious groups are at higher risk.

QUESTION 209

A diagnosis of hepatitis C is confirmed by a male client's physician.
The nurse should be knowledgeable of the differences between
hepatitis A, B, and C. Which of the following are characteristics of
hepatitis C?

A. The potential for chronic liver disease is minimal.

B. The onset of symptoms is abrupt.

C. The incubation period is 226 weeks.

D. There is an effective vaccine for hepatitis B, but not for hepatitis C.

Correct Answer: C

Explanation/Reference:

(A) Hepatitis C and B may result in chronic liver disease. Hepatitis A
has a low potential for chronic liver disease.
 (B) Hepatitis C and B have insidious onsets. Hepatitis A has an abrupt
onset.
(C) Incubation periods are as follows: hepatitis C is 226 weeks,
hepatitis B is 620 weeks, and hepatitis A is 26 weeks.
(D) Only hepatitis B has an effective vaccine.

QUESTION 210

The nurse is aware that nutrition is an important aspect of care for a
client with hepatitis. Which of the following diets would be most
therapeutic?

A. High protein and lowcarbohydrate

B. Low calorie and low protein

C. High carbohydrate and high calorie
D. Low carbohydrate and high calorie

Correct Answer: C

Explanation/Reference:

(A) Protein increases the workload of the liver. Increased
carbohydrates provide needed calories and promote palatability.
(B) Dietary intake should be adequate to ensure wound healing.
(C)Increased carbohydrates provide needed calories.
 (D) A highcalorie diet is best obtained from carbohydrates because of
their palatability. Fats increase the workload of the liver.

QUESTION 211

Which of the following nursing orders should be included in the plan of
care for a client with hepatitis C?

A. The nurse should use universal precautions when obtaining blood
    samples.
B. Total bed rest should be maintained until the client is asymptomatic.
C. The client should be instructed to maintain a low semi-Fowler
    position when eatingmeals.
D. The nurse should administer an alcohol backrub at bedtime.

Correct Answer: A

Explanation/Reference:

(A) The source of infection with hepatitis C is contaminated blood
products.
(B) Modified bed rest should be maintained while the client is
symptomatic. Routine activities can be slowly resumed once the client
is asymptomatic.
(C) Nausea and vomiting occur frequently with hepatitis C. A high
Fowler position may decrease the tendency to vomit.
(D) The buildup of bilirubin in the client's skin may cause pruritus.
Alcohol is a drying agent.

QUESTION 212

Which of the following should be included in discharge teaching for a
client with hepatitis C?

A. He should take aspirin as needed for muscle and joint pain.
B. He may become a blood donor when his liver enzymes return to
    normal.
C. He should avoid alcoholic beverages during his recovery period.
D. He should use disposable dishes for eating and drinking.

Correct Answer: C

Explanation/Reference:

(A) Aspirin is hepatotoxic, may increase bleeding, and should be
avoided.
(B) Blood should not be donated by a client who has had hepatitis C
because of the possibility of transmission of disease.
(C) Alcohol is detoxified in the liver.
(D) Hepatitis C is not spread through the oral route.

QUESTION 213

A 27-year-old man was diagnosed with type I diabetes 3 months ago.
Two weeks ago he complained of pain, redness, and tenderness in his
right lower leg. He is admitted to the hospital with a slight elevation of
temperature and vague complaints of "not feeling well." At 4:30 PM on
the day of his admission, his blood glucose level is 50 mg; dinner will
be served at 5:00 PM.

The best nursing action would be to:

A. Give him 3 tbsp of sugar dissolved in 4 oz of grape juice to drink
B. Ask him to dissolve three pieces of hard candy in his mouth
C. Have him drink 4 oz of orange juice
D. Monitor him closely until dinner arrives

Correct Answer: C

Explanation/Reference:

(A) The combination of sugar and juice will increase the blood sugar beyond the normal range.
(B) Concentrated sweets are not absorbed as fast as juice; consequently, they elevate the blood sugar beyond the normal limit.
(C) Four ounces of orange juice will act immediately to raise the blood sugar to a normal level and sustain it for 30 minutes until supper is served.
(D) There is an increased potential for the client's blood sugar to decrease even further, resulting in diabetic coma.

QUESTION 214

A male client receives 10 U of regular human insulin SC at 9:00 AM. The nurse would expect peak action from this injection to occur at:

A. 9:30 AM
B. 10:30 AM
C. 12 noon
D. 4:00 PM

Correct Answer: C

Explanation/Reference:

(A) This is too early for peak action to occur.
(B) This is too early for peak action to occur.
(C) Regular insulin peak action occurs 24 hours after administration.
(D) This is too late for peak action to occur.

QUESTION 215

A type I diabetic client is diagnosed with cellulitis in his right lower extremity. The nurse would expect which of the following to be present in relation to his blood sugar level?

A. A normal blood sugar level
B. A decreased blood sugar level

C. An increased blood sugar level

D. Fluctuating levels with a predawn increase

Correct Answer: C

Explanation/Reference:

(A) Blood sugar levels increase when the body responds to stress and illness.
(B) Blood sugar levels increase when the body responds to stress and illness.
(C) Hyperglycemia occurs because glucose is produced as the body responds to the stress and illness of cellulitis.
(D) Blood sugar levels remain elevated as long as the body responds to stress and illness.

QUESTION 216

The physician has ordered that a daily exercise program be instituted by a client with type I diabetes following his discharge from the hospital. Discharge instructions about exercise should include which of the following?

A. Exercise should be performed 30 minutes before meals.

B. A snack may be needed before and/or during exercise.

C. Hyperglycemia may occur 24 hours after exercise.

D. The blood glucose level should be 100 mg or below before exercise is begun.

Correct Answer: B

Explanation/Reference:

(A) Exercise should not be performed before meals because the blood sugar is usually lower just prior to eating; therefore, there is an increased risk for hypoglycemia.
(B) Exercise lowers blood sugar levels; therefore, a snack may be needed to maintain the appropriate glucose level.
(C) Exercise lowers blood sugar levels.
(D) Exercise lowers blood sugar levels. If the blood glucose level is 100 mg or below at the start of exercise, the potential for hypoglycemia is greater.

QUESTION 217

Dietary planning is an essential part of the diabetic client's regimen. The American Diabetes Association recommends which of the following caloric guidelines for daily meal planning?

A. 50% complex carbohydrate, 20%25% protein, 20%25% fat
B. 45% complex carbohydrate, 25%30% protein, 30%35% fat
C. 70% complex carbohydrate, 20%30% protein, 10%20% fat
D. 60% complex carbohydrate, 12%15% protein, 20%25% fat

Correct Answer: D

Explanation/Reference:

(A) The percentage of carbohydrates is too low to maintain blood sugar levels. The percent range of protein is too high and may cause extra workload on the kidney as it is metabolized.
(B) The percentage of carbohydrates is too low to maintain blood sugar levels. The percent range of protein is too high and may cause extra workload on the kidney.
(C) The percentage of carbohydrates is too high; the percent range of protein is too high, and of fat, too low.
(D) This combination provides enough carbohydrates to maintain blood glucose levels, enough protein to maintain body repair, and enough fat to ensure palatability.

QUESTION 218

A 74-year-old female client is 3 days postoperative. She has an indwelling catheter and has been progressing well. While the nurse is in the room, the client states, "Oh dear, I feel like I have to urinate again!" Which of the following is the most appropriate initial nursing response?

A. Assure her that this is most likely the result of bladder spasms.
B. Check the collection bag and tubing to verify that the catheter is draining properly.
C. Instruct her to do Kegel exercises to diminish the urge to void.
D. Ask her if she has felt this way before.

Correct Answer: B

Explanation/Reference:

(A) Although this may be an appropriate response, the initial response would be to assure the patency of the catheter.
(B) The most frequent reason for an urge to void with an indwelling catheter is blocked tubing. This response would be the best initial response.
(C) Kegel exercises while a retention catheter is in place would not help to prevent a voiding urge and could irritate the urethral sphincter.
(D) Though the nurse would want to ascertain whether the client has felt the same urge to void before, the initial response should be to assure the patency of the catheter.

QUESTION 219

In cleansing the perineal area around the site of catheter insertion, the nurse would:

A. Wipe the catheter toward the urinary meatus
B. Wipe the catheter away from the urinary meatus
C. Apply a small amount of talcum powder after drying the perineal area
D. Gently insert the catheter another 1/2 inch after cleansing to prevent irritation from the balloon

Correct Answer: B

Explanation/Reference:

(A) Wiping toward the urinary meatus would transport microorganisms from the external tubing to the urethra, thereby increasing the risk of bladder infection.
(B) Wiping away from the urinary meatus would remove microorganisms from the point of insertion of the catheter, thereby decreasing the risk of bladder infection.
(C) Talcum powder should not be applied following catheter care, because powders contribute to moisture retention and infection likelihood.
(D) The catheter should never be inserted further into the urethra, because this would serve no useful purpose and would increase the risk of infection.

QUESTION 220

Nursing interventions designed to decrease the risk of infection in a
client with an indwelling catheter include:

A. Cleanse area around the meatus twice a day
B. Empty the catheter drainage bag at least daily
C. Change the catheter tubing and bag every 48 hours
D. Maintain fluid intake of 12001500 mL every day

Correct Answer: A

Explanation/Reference:

(A) Catheter site care is to be done at least twice daily to prevent
pathogen growth at the catheter insertion site.
(B) Catheter drainage bags are usually emptied every 8 hours to
prevent urine stasis and pathogen growth.
(C) Tubing and collection bags are not changed this often, because
research studies have not demonstrated the efficacy of this practice.
(D) Fluid intake needs to be in the 20002500 mL range if possible to
help irrigate the bladder and prevent infection.

QUESTION 221

A client tells the nurse that she has had a history of urinary tract
infections. The nurse would do further health teaching if she verbalizes
she will:

A. Drink at least 8 oz of cranberry juice daily
B. Maintain a fluid intake of at least 2000 mL daily
C. Wash her hands before and after voiding
D. Limit her fluid intake after 6 PM so that there is not a great deal of
    urine in her bladder while she sleeps

Correct Answer: D

Explanation/Reference:

(A) Cranberry juice helps to maintain urine acidity, thereby retarding
bacterial growth.
(B) A generous fluid intake will help to irrigate the bladder and to
prevent bacterial growth within the bladder.

(C) Hand washing is an effective means of preventing pathogen transmission.

(D) Restricting fluid intake would contribute to urinary stasis, which in turn would contribute to bacterial growth.

QUESTION 222

An 83-year-old client has been hospitalized following a fall in his home. He has developed a possible fecal impaction. Which of the following assessment findings would be most indicative of a fecal impaction?

A. Boardlike, rigid abdomen
B. Loss of the urge to defecate
C. Liquid stool
D. Abdominal pain

Correct Answer: C

Explanation/Reference:

(A) A boardlike, rigid abdomen would point to a perforated bowel, not a fecal impaction.
(B) When a client is fecally impacted, a common symptom is the urge to defecate but the inability to do so.
(C) When an impaction is present, only liquid stool will be able to pass around the impacted site.
(D) Abdominal pain without distention is not a sign of a fecal impaction.

QUESTION 223

The nurse provides a male client with diet teaching so that he can help prevent constipation in the future. Which food choices indicate that this teaching has been understood?

A. Omelette and hash browns
B. Pancakes and syrup
C. Bagel with cream cheese
D. Cooked oatmeal and grapefruit half

Correct Answer: D

Explanation/Reference:

(A) Eggs and hash browns do not provide much fiber and bulk, so they do not effectively prevent constipation.
(B) Pancakes and syrup also have little fiber and bulk, so they do not effectively prevent constipation.
(C) Bagel and cream cheese do not provide intestinal bulk.
 (D) A combination of oatmeal and fresh fruit will provide fiber and intestinal bulk.

QUESTION 224

One of the medications that is prescribed for a male client is furosemide (Lasix) 80 mg bid. To reduce his risk of falls, the nurse would teach him to take this medication:

A. On arising and no later than 6 PM
B. At evenly spaced intervals, such as 8 AM and 8 PM
C. With at least one glass of water per pill
D. With breakfast and at bedtime

Correct Answer: A

Explanation/Reference:

(A) This option provides adequate spacing of the medication and will limit the client's need to get up to go to the bathroom during the night hours, when he is especially at high risk for falls.

(B) This option would result in the need to get up during the night to urinate and would thus increase the risk of falls. This option also does not take into consideration the client's usual daily routine.

(C) Taking this medication with at least one glass of water would not have an impact on the risk of falls.

(D) This option would result in the need to get up during the night to urinate and would thus increase the risk of falls.

QUESTION 225

The nurse teaches a male client ways to reduce the risks associated
with furosemide therapy. Which of the following indicates that he
understands this teaching?

A. "I'll be sure to rise slowly and sit for a few minutes after lying down."
B. "I'll be sure to walk at least 23 blocks every day."
C. "I'll be sure to restrict my fluid intake to four or five glasses a day."
D. "I'll be sure not to take any more aspirin while I amon this drug."

Correct Answer: A

Explanation/Reference:

(A) This response will help to prevent the occurrence of postural
hypotension, a common side effect of this drug and a common reason
for falls.
(B) Although walking is an excellent exercise, it is not specific to the
reduction of risks associated with diuretic therapy.

(C) Clients on diuretic therapy are generally taught to ensure that their
fluid intake is at least 20003000 mL daily, unless contraindicated.
(D) Aspirin is a safe drug to take along with furosemide.

QUESTION 226

A client is taught to eat foods high in potassium. Which food choices
would indicate that this teaching has been successful?

A. Pork chop, baked acorn squash, brussel sprouts
B. Chicken breast, rice, and green beans
C. Roast beef, baked potato, and diced carrots
D. Tuna casserole, noodles, and spinach

Correct Answer: A

Explanation/Reference:

(A) Both acorn squash and brussels sprouts are potassium-rich foods.
(B) None of these foods is considered potassium rich.

(C) Only the baked potato is a potassium-rich food.
(D) Spinach is the only potassium-rich food in this option.

QUESTION 227

The nurse would be sure to instruct a client on the signs and
symptoms of an eye infection and hemorrhage. These signs and
symptoms would include:

A. Blurred vision and dizziness
B. Eye pain and itching
C. Feeling of eye pressure and headache
D. Eye discharge and hemoptysis

Correct Answer: B

Explanation/Reference:

(A) Although blurred vision may occur, dizziness would not be
    associated with an infection or hemorrhage.
(B) Eye pain is a symptom of hemorrhage within the eye, and itching is
associated with infection.

(C) Nausea and headache would not be usual symptoms of eye
    hemorrhage or infection.
(D) Some eye discharge might be anticipated if an infection is present;
hemoptysis would not.

QUESTION 228

The nurse would teach a male client ways to minimize the risk of
infection after eye surgery. Which of the following indicates the client
needs further teaching?

A. "I will wash my hands before instilling eye medications."
B. "I will wear sunglasses when going outside."
C. "I will wear an eye patch for the first 3 postoperative days."
D. "I will maintain the sterility of the eye medications."

Correct Answer: C

Explanation/Reference:

(A) Hand washing would be an important action designed to prevent transmission of pathogens from the hands to the eye.
(B) Wearing sunglasses when going outside will prevent airborne pathogens from entering the eye.
(C) Eye patches are most frequently ordered to be worn while the client sleeps or naps, not constantly for this length of time.
(D) Eye medications are sterile; clients need to be taught how to maintain this sterility.

QUESTION 229

With a geriatric client, the nurse should also assess whether he has been obtaining a yearly vaccination against influenza. Why is this assessment important?

A. Influenza is growing in our society.
B. Older clients generally are sicker than others when stricken with flu.
C. Older clients have less effective immune systems.
D. Older clients have more exposure to the causative agents.

Correct Answer: C

Explanation/Reference:

(A) Although influenza is common, the elderly are more at risk because of decreased effectiveness of their immune system, not because the incidence is increasing.
(B) Older clients have the same degree of illness when stricken as other populations.
(C) As people age, their immune system becomes less effective, increasing their risk for influenza.
(D) Older clients have no more exposure to the causative agents than do school-age children, for example.

QUESTION 230

In evaluating the laboratory results of a client with severe pressure ulcers, the nurse finds that her albumin level is low. A decrease in serum albumin would contribute to the formation of pressure ulcers because:

A. The proteins needed for tissue repair are diminished.
B. The iron stores needed for tissue repair are inadequate.
C. A decreased serum albumin level indicates kidney disease.
D. A decreased serum albumin causes fluid movement into the blood vessels, causing dehydration.

Correct Answer: A

Explanation/Reference:

(A) Serum albumin levels indicate the adequacy of protein stores available for tissue repair.
(B) Serum albumin does not measure iron stores.
(C) Serum albumin levels do not measure kidneyfunction.
(D) A decreased serum albumin level would cause fluid movement out of blood vessels, not into them.

QUESTION 231

Which of the following menu choices would indicate that a client with pressure ulcers understands the role diet plays in restoring her albumin levels?

A. Broiled fish with rice
B. Bran flakes with fresh peaches
C. Lasagna with garlic bread
D. Cauliflower and lettuce salad

Correct Answer: A

Explanation/Reference:

(A) Broiled fish and rice are both excellent sources of protein.
(B) Fresh fruits are not a good source of protein.
(C) Foods in the bread group are not high in protein.
(D) Most vegetables are not high in protein; peas and beans are the major vegetables higher in protein.

QUESTION 232

The nurse observes that a client has difficulty chewing and swallowing her food. A nursing response designed to reduce this problem would include:

A. Ordering a full liquid diet for her
B. Ordering five small meals for her
C. Ordering a mechanical soft diet for her
D. Ordering a puréed diet for her

Correct Answer: C

Explanation/Reference:

(A) Full liquids would be difficult to swallow if the muscle control of the swallowing act is affected; this is a probable reason for her difficulties, given her medical diagnosis of multiple sclerosis.
(B) Five small meals would do little if anything to decrease her swallowing difficulties, other than assure that she tires less easily.
(C) A mechanical soft diet should be easier to chew and swallow, because foods would be more evenly consistent.
(D) A pureed diet would cause her to regress more than might be needed; the mechanical soft diet should be tried first.

QUESTION 233

When a client with pancreatitis is discharged, the nurse needs to teach him how to prevent another occurrence of acute pancreatitis. Which of the following statements would indicate he has an understanding of his disease?

A. "I will not eat any raw or uncooked vegetables."
B. "I will limit my alcohol to one cocktail per day."

C. "I will look into attending Alcoholics Anonymous meetings."

D. "I will report any changes in bowel movements to my doctor."

Correct Answer: C

Explanation/Reference:

(A) Raw or uncooked vegetables are all right to eat postdischarge.

(B) This client must avoid any alcohol intake.

(C) The client displays awareness of the need to avoid alcohol.

(D) This action would be pertinent only if fatty stools associated with chronic hepatitis were the problem.

QUESTION 234

A 54-year-old client is admitted to the hospital with a possible gastric ulcer. He is a heavy smoker. When discussing his smoking habits with him, the nurse should advise him to:

A. Smoke low-tar, filtered cigarettes

B. Smoke cigars instead

C. Smoke only right after meals

D. Chew gum instead

Correct Answer: C

Explanation/Reference:

(A, B, D) Cigarettes, cigars, and chewing gum would stimulate gastric acid secretion.

(C) Smoking on a full stomach minimizes effect of nicotine on gastric acid.

QUESTION 235

Iron dextran (Imferon) is a parenteral iron preparation. The nurse should know that it:

A. Is also called intrinsic factor

B. Must be given in the abdomen

C. Requires use of the Z-track method

D. Should be given SC

Correct Answer: C

Explanation/Reference:

(A) Intrinsic factor is needed to absorb vitamin B12.
(B) Iron dextran is given parenterally, but Z-track in a large muscle.
(C) A Ztrack method of injection is required to prevent staining and irritation of the tissue.
(D) An SC injection is not deep enough and may cause subcutaneous fat abscess formation.

QUESTION 236

A nasogastric (NG) tube inserted preoperatively is attached to low, intermittent suctions. A client with an NG tube exhibits these symptoms: He is restless; serum electrolytes are Na 138, K 4.0, blood pH 7.53. This client is most likely experiencing:

A. Hyperkalemia

B. Hyponatremia

C. Metabolic acidosis

D. Metabolic alkalosis

Correct Answer: D

Explanation/Reference:

(A) Sodium level is within normal limits.
(B) Sodium level is within normal limits.
(C) pH level is consistent with alkalosis.
(D) With an NG tube attached to low, intermittent suction, acids are removed and a client will develop metabolic alkalosis.

QUESTION 237

A client is experiencing muscle weakness and lethargy. His serum K+is 3.2. What other symptoms might he exhibit?

A. Tetany
B. Dysrhythmias
C. Numbness of extremities
D. Headache

Correct Answer: B

Explanation/Reference:

(A) Tetany is seen with low calcium.
(B) Low potassium causes dysrhythmias because potassium is responsible for cardiac muscle activity.
(C) Numbness of extremities is seen with high potassium.
(D) Headache is not associated with potassium excess or deficiency.

QUESTION 238

Following a gastric resection, which of the following actions would the nurse reinforce with the client in order to alleviate the distress from dumping syndrome?

A. Eating three large meals a day
B. Drinking small amounts of liquids with meals
C. Taking a long walk after meals
D. Eating a low-carbohydrate diet

Correct Answer: D

Explanation/Reference:

(A) Six small meals are recommended.
(B) Liquids after meals increase the time food empties from the stomach.
(C) Lying down after meals is recommended to prevent gravity from producing dumping.
(D) A low-carbohydrate diet will prevent a hypertonic bolus, which causes dumping.

QUESTION 239

Azulfidine (Sulfasalazine) may be ordered for a client who has
ulcerative colitis. Which of the following is a nursing implication for this
drug?

A. Limit fluids to 500 mL/day.
B. Administer 2 hours before meals.
C. Observe for skin rash and diarrhea.
D. Monitor blood pressure, pulse.

Correct Answer: C

Explanation/Reference:

(A) Fluids up to 25003000 mL/day are needed to prevent kidney
stones.
(B) The client should be instructed to take oral preparations with meals
or snacks to lessen gastric irritation.
(C) Sulfasalazine causes skin rash and diarrhea.
(D) Blood pressure and pulse are not altered by sulfasalazine.

QUESTION 240

Other drugs may be ordered to manage a client's ulcerative colitis.
Which of the following medications, if ordered, would the nurse
question?

A. Methylprednisolone sodium succinate (Solu-Medrol)
B. Loperamide (Imodium)
C. Psyllium
D. 6-Mercaptopurine

Correct Answer: D

Explanation/Reference:

(A) Methylprednisolone sodium succinate is used for its anti-
inflammatory effects.
(B) Loperamide would be used to control diarrhea.

(C) Psyllium may improve consistency of stools by providing bulk.
(D) An immunosuppressant such as 6-mercaptopurine is used for chronic unrelenting Crohn's disease.

QUESTION 241

A male client is scheduled for a liver biopsy. In preparing him for this test, the nurse should:

A. Explain that he will be kept NPO for 24 hours before the exam
B. Practice with him so he will be able to hold his breath for 1 minute
C. Explain that he will be receiving a laxative to prevent a distended bowel from applying pressure on the liver
D. Explain that his vital signs will be checked frequently after the test

Correct Answer: D

Explanation/Reference:

(A) There is no NPO restriction prior to a liver biopsy.
(B) The client would need to hold his breath for 510 seconds.
(C) There is no pretest laxative given.
(D) Following the test, the client is watched for hemorrhage and shock.

QUESTION 242

After a liver biopsy, the best position for the client is:

A. High Fowler
B. Prone
C. Supine
D. Right lateral

Correct Answer: D

Explanation/Reference:

(A) This position does not help to prevent bleeding.
(B) This position does not help to prevent bleeding.
(C) This position does not help to prevent bleeding.
(D) The right lateral position would allow pressure on the liver to prevent bleeding.

QUESTION 243

A complication for which the nurse should be alert following a liver biopsy is:

A. Hepatic coma
B. Jaundice
C. Ascites
D. Shock

Correct Answer: D

Explanation/Reference:

(A) Hepatic coma may occur in liver disease due to the increased NH3levels, not due to liver biopsy.
(B) Jaundice may occur due to increased bilirubin levels, not due to liver biopsy.
(C) Ascites would occur due to portal hypertension, not due to liver biopsy.
(D) Hemorrhage and shock are the most likely complications after liver biopsy because of already existing bleeding tendencies in the vascular makeup of the liver.

QUESTION 244

Which nursing implication is appropriate for a client undergoing a paracentesis?

A. Have the client void before the procedure.
B. Keep the client NPO.
C. Observe the client for hypertension following the procedure.
D. Place the client on the right side following the procedure.

Correct Answer: A

Explanation/Reference:

(A) A full bladder would impede withdrawal of ascitic fluid. (B) Keeping the client NPO is not necessary.
(C) The client may exhibit signs and symptoms of shock and hypertension.
(D) No position change is needed after the procedure.

QUESTION 245

The nurse would assess the client's correct understanding of the fertility awareness methods that enhance conception, if the client stated that:

A. "My sexual partner and I should have intercourse when my cervical mucosa is thick and cloudy."
B. "At ovulation, my basal body temperature should rise about 0.5F."
C. "I should douche immediately after intercourse."
D. "My sexual partner and I should have sexual intercourse on day 14 of my cycle regardless of the length

   of the cycle."

Correct Answer: B

Explanation/Reference:

(A) At ovulation, the cervical mucus is increased, stretchable, and watery clear.
(B) Under the influence of progesterone, the basal body temperature increases slightly after ovulation.
(C) To enhance fertility, measures should be taken that promote retention of sperm rather than removal.
(D) Ovulation, the optimal time for conception, occurs 14+2 days before the next menses; therefore, the date of ovulation is directly related to the length of the menstrual cycle.

QUESTION 246

A couple is planning the conception of their first child. The wife, whose normal menstrual cycle is 34 days in length, correctly identifies the time that she is most likely to ovulate if she states that ovulation should occur on day:

A. 14+2 days
B. 16+2 days
C. 20+2 days
D. 22+2 days

Correct Answer: C

Explanation/Reference:

(A) Ovulation is dependent on average length of menstrual cycle, not standard 14 days.
(B) Ovulation occurs 14+2 days before next menses (34 minus 14 does not equal 16).
(C) Ovulation occurs 14+2 days before next menses (34 minus 14 equals 20).
(D) Ovulation occurs 14+2 days before next menses (34 minus 14 does not equal 22).

QUESTION 247

A client is pregnant with her second child. Her last menstrual period began on January 15. Her expected date of delivery would be:

A. October 8
B. October 15
C. October 22
D. October 29

Correct Answer: C

Explanation/Reference:

(A) Incorrect application of Nägele's rule: correctly subtracted 3 months but subtracted 7 days rather than added.
(B) Incorrect application of Nägele's rule: correctly subtracted 3 months but did not add 7 days.

(C) Correct application of Nägele's rule: correctly subtracted 3 months and added 7 days.
(D) Incorrect application of Nägele's rule: correctly subtracted 3 months but added 14 days instead of 7 days.

QUESTION 248

The nurse instructs a pregnant client (G2P1) to rest in a side-lying position and avoid lying flat on her back. The nurse explains that this is to avoid "vena caval syndrome," a condition which:

A. Occurs when blood pressure increases sharply with changes in position
B. Results when blood flow from the extremities is blocked or slowed
C. Is seen mainly in first pregnancies
D. May require medication if positioning does not help

Correct Answer: B

Explanation/Reference:

(A) Blood pressure changes are predominantly due to pressure of the gravid uterus.
(B) Pressure of the gravid uterus on the inferior vena cava decreases blood return from lower extremities.
(C) Inferior vena cava syndrome is experienced in the latter months of pregnancy regardless of parity.
(D) There are no medications useful in the treatment of interior vena cava syndrome; alleviating pressure by position changes is effective.

QUESTION 249

A pregnant client comes to the office for her first prenatal examination at 10 weeks. She has been pregnant twice before; the first delivery produced a viable baby girl at 39 weeks 3 years ago; the second pregnancy produced a viable baby boy at 36 weeks 2 years ago. Both children are living and well. Using the GTPAL system to record her obstetrical history, the nurse should record:

A. 3-2-0-0-2
B. 2-2-0-2-2
C. 3-1-1-0-2
D. 2-1-1-0-2

Correct Answer: C

Explanation/Reference:

(A) This answer is an incorrect application of the GTPAL method. One prior pregnancy was a preterm birth at 36 weeks (T =1, P= 1; not T = 2).
(B) This answer is an incorrect application of the GTPAL method. The client is currently pregnant for the third time (G = 3, not 2), one prior pregnancy was preterm (T= 1, P= 1; not T= 2), and she has had no prior abortions (A =0).
(C) This answer is the correct application of GTPAL method. The client is currently pregnant for the third time (G =3), her first pregnancy ended at term (>37 weeks) (T =1), her second pregnancy ended preterm 2033 weeks) (P = 1), she has no history of abortion (A =0), and she has two living children (L = 2).
(D) This answer is an incorrect application of the GTPAL method. The client is currently pregnant for the third time (G =3, not 2).

QUESTION 250

A pregnant client comes to the office for her first prenatal examination at 10 weeks. She has been pregnant twice before; the first delivery produced a viable baby girl at 39 weeks 3 years ago; the second pregnancy produced a viable baby boy at 36 weeks 2 years ago. Both children are living and well. Using the gravida and para system to record the client's obstetrical history, the nurse should record:

A. Gravida 3 para 1
B. Gravida 3 para 2
C. Gravida 2 para 1
D. Gravida 2 para 2

Correct Answer: B

Explanation/Reference:

(A) This answer is an incorrect application of gravida and para. The client has had two prior deliveries of more than 20 weeks' gestation; therefore, para equals 2, not 1.
(B) This answer is the correct application of gravida and para. The client is currently pregnant for the third time (G = 3), regardless of the length of the pregnancy, and has had two prior pregnancies with birth after the 20th week (P = 2), whether infant was alive or dead.

(C) This answer is an incorrect application of gravida and para. The client is currently pregnant for the third time (G = 3, not 2); prior pregnancies lasted longer than 20 weeks (therefore, P = 2, not 1).
(D) This is an incorrect application of gravida and para. Client is currently pregnant for third time (G
= 3, not 2).

QUESTION 251

A gravida 2 para 1 client is hospitalized with severe preeclampsia. While she receives magnesium sulfate (MgSO4) therapy, the nurse knows it is safe to repeat the dosage if:

A. Deep tendon reflexes are absent
B. Urine output is 20 mL/hr
C. MgSO4serum levels are>15 mg/dL
D. Respirations are>16 breaths/min

Correct Answer: D

Explanation/Reference:

(A) MgSO4is a central nervous system depressant. Loss of reflexes is often the first sign of developing toxicity.
(B) Urinary output at <25 mL/hr or 100 mL in 4 hours may result in the accumulation of toxic levels of magnesium.
(C) The therapeutic serum range for MgSO4is 68 mg/dL. Higher levels indicate toxicity.
(D) Respirations of>16 breaths/min indicate that toxic levels of magnesium have not been reached. Medication administration would be safe.

QUESTION 252

Prenatal clients are routinely monitored for early signs of pregnancy-induced hypertension (PIH). For the prenatal client, which of the following blood pressure changes from baseline would be most significant for the nurse to report as indicative of PIH?

A. 136/88 to 144/93
B. 132/78 to 124/76

C. 114/70 to 140/88
D. 140/90 to 148/98

Correct Answer: C

Explanation/Reference:

(A) These blood pressure changes reflect only an 8 mm Hg systolic and a 5 mm Hg diastolic increase, which is insufficient for blood pressure changes indicating PIH.
(B) These bloodpressure changes reflect a decrease in systolic pressure of 8 mm Hg and diastolic pressure of 2 mm Hg; these values are not indicative of blood pressure increases reflecting PIH. (C) The definition of PIH is an increase in systolic blood pressure of 30 mm Hg and/or diastolic blood pressure of 15 mm Hg. These blood pressures reflect a change of 26 mm Hg systolically and 18 mm Hg diastolically. (D) These blood pressures reflect a change of only 8 mm Hg systolically and 8 mm Hg diastolically, which is insufficient for blood pressure changes indicating PIH.

QUESTION 253

In assisting preconceptual clients, the nurse should teach that the corpus luteum secretes progesterone,

which thickens the endometrial lining in which of the phases of the menstrual cycle?

A. Menstrual phase
B. Proliferative phase
C. Secretory phase
D. Ischemic phase

Correct Answer: C

Explanation/Reference:

(A) Menses occurs during the menstrual phase, during which levels of both estrogen and progesterone are decreased.
(B) The ovarian hormone responsible for the proliferative phase, during which the uterine endometrium enlarges, is estrogen.

(C) The ovarian hormone responsible for the secretory phase is
progesterone, which is secreted by the corpus luteum and causes
marked swelling in the uterine endometrium.
(D) The corpus luteum begins to degenerate in the ischemic phase,
causing a fall in both estrogen and progesterone.

QUESTION 254

A client decided early in her pregnancy to breast-feed her first baby.
She gave birth to a normal, full- term girl and is now progressing toward
the establishment of successful lactation. To remove the baby from her
breast, she should be instructed to:

A. Gently pull the infant away
B. Withdraw the breast from the infant's mouth
C. Compress the areolar tissue until the infant drops the nipple from
    her mouth
D. Insert a clean finger into the baby's mouth beside the nipple

Correct Answer: D

Explanation/Reference:

(A) In pulling the infant away from the breast without breaking suction,
nipple trauma is likely to occur.
(B) In pulling the breast away from the infant without breaking suction,
nipple trauma is likely to occur.
(C) Compressing the maternal tissue does not break the suction of the
infant on the breast and can cause nipple trauma.
(D) By inserting a finger into the infant's mouth beside the nipple, the
lactating mother can break the suction and the nipple can be removed
without trauma.

QUESTION 255

A gravida 2 para 1 client delivered a full-term newborn 12 hours ago.
The nurse finds her uterus to be boggy, high, and deviated to the right.
The most appropriate nursing action is to:

A. Notify the physician
B. Place the client on a pad count
C.

D. Massage the uterus and re-evaluate in 30 minutes

E. Have the client void and then re-evaluate the fundus

Correct Answer: D

Explanation/Reference:

(A) The nurse should initiate actions to remove the most frequent cause of uterine displacement, which

involves emptying the bladder. Notifying the physician is an inappropriate nursing action.

(B) The pad count gives an estimate of blood loss, which is likely to increase with a boggy uterus; but this action does not remove the most frequent cause of uterine displacement, which is a full bladder.

(C) Massage may firm the uterus temporarily, but if a full bladder is not emptied,the uterus will remain displaced and is likely to relax again.

(D) The most common cause of uterine displacement is a full bladder.

QUESTION 256

A client delivered her first-born son 4 hours ago. She asks the nurse what the white cheeselike substance is under the baby's arms. The nurse should respond:

A. "This is a normal skin variation in newborns. It will go away in a few days."
B. "Let me have a closer look at it. The baby may have an infection."
C. "This material, called vernix, covered the baby before it was born. It will disappear in a few days."
D. "Babies sometimes have sebaceous glands that get plugged at birth. This substance is an example of that condition."

Correct Answer: C

Explanation/Reference:

(A) This response identifies the fact that vernix is a normal neonatal variation, but it does not teach the client medical terms that may be useful in understanding other healthcare personnel.
(B) This response may raise maternal anxiety and incorrectly identifies a normal neonatal variation.

(C) This response correctly identifies this neonatal variation and helps the client to understand medical terms as well as the characteristics of her newborn.
(D) Blocked sebaceous glands produce milia, particularly present on the nose.

QUESTION 257

A client is in early labor. Her fetus is in a left occipitoanterior (LOA) position; fetal heart sounds are best auscultated just:

A. Below the umbilicus toward left side of mother's abdomen
B. Below the umbilicus toward right side of mother's abdomen
C. At the umbilicus
D. Above the umbilicus to the left side of mother's abdomen

Correct Answer: A

Explanation/Reference:

(A) LOA identifies a fetus whose back is on its mother's left side, whose head is the presenting part, and whose back is toward its mother's anterior. It is easiest to auscultate fetal heart tones (FHTs) through the fetus's back.
(B) The identified fetus's back is on its mother's left side, not right side. It is easiest to auscultate FHTs through the fetus's back.
(C) In an LOA position, the fetus's head is presenting with the back to the left anterior side of the mother. The umbilicus is too high of a landmark for auscultating the fetus's heart rate through its back.
(D) This is the correct auscultation point for a fetus in the left sacroanterior position, where the sacrum is presenting, not LOA.

QUESTION 258

In performing the initial nursing assessment on a client at the prenatal clinic, the nurse will know that which of the following alterations is abnormal during pregnancy?

A. Striae gravidarum
B. Chloasma
C. Dysuria
D. Colostrum

Correct Answer: C

Explanation/Reference:

(A) Striae gravidarum are the normal stretch marks that frequently occur on the breasts, abdomen, and thighs as pregnancy progresses.
(B) Chloasma is the "mask of pregnancy" that normally occurs in many pregnant women.
(C) Dysuria is an abnormal danger sign during pregnancy and may indicate a urinary tract infection.
(D) Colostrum is a yellow breast secretion that is normally present during the last trimester of pregnancy.

QUESTION 259

A 35-weeks-pregnant client is undergoing a nonstress test (NST). During the 20-minute examination, the nurse notes three fetal movements accompanied by accelerations of the fetal heart rate, each 15 bpm, lasting 15 seconds. The nurse interprets this test to be:

A. Nonreactive
B. Reactive
C. Positive
D. Negative

Correct Answer: B

Explanation/Reference:

(A) In a nonreactive NST, the criteria for reactivity are not met.
(B) A reactive NST shows at least two accelerations of FHR with fetal movements, each 15 bpm, lasting 15 seconds or more, over 20 minutes.
(C, D) This term is used to interpret a contraction stress test (CST), or oxytocin challenge test, not an NST.

QUESTION 260

The nurse is caring for a laboring client. Assessment data include cervical dilation 9 cm; contractions every 12 minutes; strong, large amount of "bloody show." The most appropriate nursing goal for this client would be:

A. Maintain client's privacy.
B. Assist with assessment procedures.
C. Provide strategies to maintain client control.
D. Enlist additional caregiver support to ensure client's safety.

Correct Answer: C

Explanation/Reference:

(A) Privacy may help the laboring client feel safer, but measures that enhance coping take priority.
(B) The frequency of assessments do increase in transition, but helping the client to maintain control and cope with this phase of labor takes on importance.

(C) This laboring client is in transition, the most difficult part of the first stage of labor because of decreased frequency, increased duration and intensity, and decreased resting phase of the uterine contraction. The client's ability to cope is most threatened during this phase of labor, and nursing actions are directed toward helping the client to maintain control.
(D) Safety is a concern throughout labor, but helping the client to cope takes on importance in transition.

QUESTION 261

A client is admitted to the labor unit. On vaginal examination, the presenting part in a cephalic presentation was at station plus two. Station 12 means that the:

A. Presenting part is 2 cm above the level of the ischial spines
B. Biparietal diameter is at the level of the ischial spines
C. Presenting part is 2 cm below the level of the ischial spines
D. Biparietal diameter is 5 cm above the ischial spines

Correct Answer: C

Explanation/Reference:

(A) Station is the relationship of the presenting part to an imaginary line drawn between the ischial spines. If the presenting part is above the ischial spines, the station is negative. (B) When the biparietal diameter is at the level of the ischial spines, the presenting part is generally at a +4 or +5 station. (C) Station is the relationship of the presenting part to an imaginary line drawn between the ischial spines. If the presenting part is below the ischial spines, the station is positive. Thus, 2 cm below the ischial spines is the station +2.
(D) When the biparietal diameter is above the ischial spines by 5 cm, the presenting part is usually engaged or at station 0.

QUESTION 262

A pregnant client is at the clinic for a third trimester prenatal visit. During this examination, it has been determined that her fetus is in a vertex presentation with the occiput located in her right anterior quadrant. On her chart this would be noted as:

A. Right occipitoposterior
B. Right occipitoanterior
C. Right sacroanterior
D. LOA

Correct Answer: B

Explanation/Reference:

(A) The fetus in the right occipitoposterior position would be presenting with the occiput in the maternal right posterior quadrant. (B) Fetal position is defined by the location of the fetal presenting part in the four quadrants of the maternal pelvis. The right occipitoanterior is a fetus presenting with the occiput in mother's right anterior quadrant. (C) The fetus in right sacroanterior position would be presenting a sacrum, not an occiput. (D) The fetus in left occipitoanterior position would be presenting with the occiput in the mother's left anterior quadrant.

QUESTION 263

Assessment of parturient reveals the following: cervical dilation 6 cm and station 22; no progress in the last 4 hours. Uterine contractions decreasing in frequency and intensity. Marked molding of the presenting fetal head is described. The physician orders, "Begin oxytocin induction at 1 mU/min." The nurse should:

A. Begin the oxytocin induction as ordered
B. Increase the dosage by 2 mU/min increments at15-minute intervals
C. Maintain the dosage when duration of contractions is 4060 seconds and frequency is at 21/24 minute intervals
D. Question the order

Correct Answer: D

Explanation/Reference:

(A) Oxytocin stimulates labor but should not be used until CPD (cephalopelvic disproportion) is ruled out in a dysfunctional labor. (B) This answer is the correct protocol for oxytocin administration, but the medication should not be used until CPD is ruled out. (C) This answer is the correct manner to interpret effective stimulation, but oxytocin should not be used until CPD is ruled out. (D) This answer is the appropriate nursing action because the scenario presents a dysfunctional labor pattern that may be caused by CPD. Oxytocin administration is contraindicated in CPD.

QUESTION 264

A client in active labor asks the nurse for coaching with her breathing during contractions. The client has attended Lamaze birth preparation classes. Which of the following is the best response by the nurse?
A. "Keep breathing with your abdominal muscles as long as you can."

B. "Make sure you take a deep cleansing breath as the contractions start, focus on an object, and breathe about 1620 times a minute with shallow chest breaths."
C. "Find a comfortable position before you start a contraction. Once the contraction has started, take slow breaths using your abdominal muscles."

D. "If a woman in labor listens to her body and takes rapid, deep breaths, she will be able to deal with her contractions quite well."

Correct Answer: B

Explanation/Reference:

(A) Lamaze childbirth preparation teaches the use of chest, not abdominal, breathing. (B) In Lamaze preparation, every patterned breath is preceded by a cleansing breath; as labor progresses, shallow, paced breathing is found to be effective. (C) It is important to assume a comfortable position in labor, but the Lamazeprepared laboring woman is taught to breathe with her chest, not abdominal, muscles. (D) When deep chest breathing patterns are used in Lamaze preparation, they are slowly paced at a rate of 69 breaths/min.

QUESTION 265

A client is being discharged and will continue enteral feedings at home. Which of the following statements by a family member indicates the need for further teaching?

A. "If he develops diarrhea lasting for more than 23 days, I will contact thedoctor or nurse."
B. "I should anticipate that he will gain about 1 lb/day now that he is on continuous feedings."
C. "It is important to keep the head of his bed elevated or sit him in the chair duringfeedings."
D. "I should use prepared or open formula within 24 hours and store unused portions in the refrigerator."

Correct Answer: B

Explanation/Reference:

(A) Diarrhea is a complication of tube feedings that can lead to dehydration. Diarrhea may be the result of hypertonic formulas that can draw fluid into the bowel. Other causes of diarrhea may be bacterial contamination, fecal impaction, medications, and low albumin.
(B) A consistent weight gain of more than 0.22 kg/day (1/2 lb/day) over several days should be reported promptly. The client should be evaluated for fluid volume excess
(C) Elevating the client's head prevents reflux and thus formula from entering the airway.
(D) Bacteria proliferate rapidly in enteral formulas and can cause gastroenteritis and even sepsis.

QUESTION 266

A 74-year-old obese man who has undergone open reduction and internal fixation of the right hip is 8 days postoperative. He has a history of arthritis and atrial fibrillation. He admits to right lower leg pain, described as "a cramp in my leg." An appropriate nursing action is to:

A. Assess for pain with plantiflexion
B. Assess for edema and heat of the right leg
C. Instruct him to rub the cramp out of his leg
D. Elevate right lower extremity with pillows propped under the knee

Correct Answer: B

Explanation/Reference:

(A) Calf pain with dorsiflexion of the foot (Homans' sign) can be a sign of a deep venous thrombosis; however, it is not diagnostic of the condition.
(B) Swelling and warmth along the affected vein are commonly observed clinical manifestations of a deep venous thrombosis as a result of inflammation of the vessel wall.
(C) Rubbing or massaging of the affected leg is contraindicated because of the risk of the clot breaking loose and becoming an embolus.
(D) A pillow behind the knee can be constricting and further impair blood flow.

QUESTION 267

A male client is started on IV anticoagulant therapy with heparin. Which of the following laboratory studies will be ordered to monitor the therapeutic effects of heparin?

A. Partial thromboplastin time
B. Hemoglobin
C. Red blood cell (RBC) count
D. Prothrombin time

Correct Answer: A

Explanation/Reference:

(A) Partial thromboplastin time is used to monitor the effects of heparin, and dosage is adjusted depending on test results. It is a screening test used to detect deficiencies in all plasma clotting factors except factors VII and XIII and platelets.
(B) Hemoglobin is the main component of RBCs. Its main function is to carry O2from the lungs to the body tissues and to transport CO2back to the lungs.
(C) RBC count is the determination of the number of RBCs found in each cubic millimeter of whole blood.
(D) PT is used to monitor the effects of oral anticoagulants, e.g., coumarintype anticoagulants.

QUESTION 268

A client with stress incontinence should be advised:

A. to purchase absorbent undergarments.
B. that Kegel exercises might help.
C. that effective surgical treatments are nonexistent.
D. that behavioral therapy is ineffective.

Correct Answer: B

Explanation/Reference:

Kegel exercises, tightening and releasing the pelvic floor muscles, might improve stress incontinence.
Choice 1 is not an appropriate treatment for stress incontinence.
Several effective surgical treatments exist.
Lifestyle and dietary modifications can also be helpful. Physiological Adaptation

QUESTION 269

An appropriate intervention for the client with suspected genitourinary trauma and visible blood at the urethral meatus is:

A. insertion of a Foley catheter.
B. in and out catheter specimen for urinalysis.
C. a voided urine specimen for urinalysis.
D. a urologist consult.

Correct Answer: D

Explanation/Reference:

A urologist consult is appropriate for a client with visible blood at the urethral meatus and suspected trauma.
Choices 1 and 2 are contraindicated. A urinalysis might be ordered by the physician, but the question does not provide enough information to make Choice 3 the correct answer. Physiological Adaptation

QUESTION 270

Erythropoietin used to treat anemia in clients with renal failure should be given in conjunction with:

A. iron, folic acid, and B12.
B. an increase of protein in the diet.
C. vitamins A and C.
D. an increase of calcium in the diet.

Correct Answer: A

Explanation/Reference:

The kidneys of a client in renal failure produce no erythropoietin, a hormone necessary for RBC production. Erythropoietin can be given as replacement, but the client needs adequate iron, folate, and B12 to increase the effectiveness of EPO. Choice 2 is not necessary for RBC production and can increase uremia. Choices 3 and 4 are not necessary for RBC production.Physiological Adaptation

QUESTION 271

The kind of man who beats a woman is:

A. from a minority culture in a low-income group.
B. from a majority culture in a middle-income group.
C. one who was never allowed to compete as a child.
D. from any walk of life, race, income group, or profession.

Correct Answer: D

Explanation/Reference:

Batterers cannot be predicted by demographic features related to age, ethnicity, race, religious denomination, education, socioeconomic status, or class. Ninety-five percent of domestic abuse cases involve male perpetrators and female victims. Psychosocial Integrity

QUESTION 272

A batterer is usually someone who:

A. grew up in a loving, secure home.
B. was an only child.
C. was physically or psychologically abused.
D. admits he has a problem with anger.

Correct Answer: C

Explanation/Reference:

Many batterers report having been abused as children. Psychosocial Integrity

QUESTION 273

When helping a client gain insight into anxiety, the nurse should:

A. help relate anxiety to specific behaviors.
B. ask the client to describe events that precede increased anxiety.
C. instruct the client to practice relaxation techniques.
D. confront the client's resistive behavior.

Correct Answer: B

Explanation/Reference:

To gain insight, the client needs to recognize causal events. The other activities focus on recognition of anxiety. Psychosocial Integrity

QUESTION 274

What interpersonal relief behavior is Ashley using?

A. acting out
B. somatizing
C. withdrawal
D. problem-solving

Correct Answer: B

Explanation/Reference:

Somatizing means one experiences an emotional conflict as a physical symptom. Ashley manifests several physical symptoms associated with severe anxiety. Acting out refers to behaviors such as anger, crying, laughter, and physical or verbal abuse. Withdrawal is a reaction in which psychic energy is withdrawn from the environment and focused on the self in response to anxiety. Problem-solving takes place when anxiety is identified and the unmet need is met. Psychosocial Integrity

QUESTION 275

A primary belief of psychiatric mental health nursing is:

A. most people have the potential to change and grow.
B. every person is worthy of dignity and respect.
C. human needs are individual to each person.
D. some behaviors have no meaning and cannot be understood.

Correct Answer: B

Explanation/Reference:

Every person is worthy of dignity and respect. Every person has the potential to change and grow. All people have basic human needs in common with others. All behavior has meaning and can be understood from the client's perspective.Psychosocial Integrity

QUESTION 276

James returns home from school angry and upset because his teacher gave him a low grade on an assignment. After returning home from school, he kicks the dog. This coping mechanism is known as:

A. denial.
B. suppression.
C. displacement.
D. fantasy.

Correct Answer: C

Explanation/Reference:

Displacement is the transference of anger to another. Anger is displaced on the dog as a convenient object.
Psychosocial Integrity

QUESTION 277

A woman asks, "How much alcohol can I safely drink while pregnant?"
The nurse's best response is:

A. "The amount of alcohol that is safe during pregnancy is unknown."
B. "Consuming one or two beers or glasses of wine a day is
    considered safe for a healthy pregnant woman."
C. "Drinking three or more drinks on any given occasion is the only
    harmful type of drinking during pregnancy."
D. "You can have a drink to help you relax and get to sleep at night."

Correct Answer: A

Explanation/Reference:

The amount of alcohol that is safe during pregnancy is unknown. Fetal
alcohol syndrome is a combination of mental and physical
abnormalities present in infants born to mothers who have consumed
alcohol during pregnancy. Psychosocial Integrity

QUESTION 278

A client is taking hydrocodone (Vicodin) for chronic back pain. The
client has required an increase in the dose and asks whether this
means he is addicted to Vicodin. The nurse should base her reply on
the knowledge that:

A. the client's body has developed tolerance, requiring more drug to
    produce the same effect.
B. the client is preoccupied with getting the drug and is experiencing
    loss of control, indicating drug dependence.
C. addiction is the term used to describe physical dependence with
    withdrawal symptoms and tolerance.
D. the client has a dual diagnosis of substance abuse and chronic
    back pain.

Correct Answer: A

Drug tolerance is characterized by the ability to ingest a larger dose without adverse effect and decreased sensitivity to the substance. Substance dependence is a severe condition indicating physical problems and disruption of the person's social, family, and work life. The psychological behaviors related to substance use are termed addiction. Dual diagnosis is the coexistence of substance abuse and psychiatric disorders. Psychosocial Integrity

QUESTION 279

Which is the proper hand position for performing chest percussion?

A. cup the hands
B. use the side of the hands
C. flatten the hands
D. spread the fingers of both hands

Correct Answer: A

The hands are cupped for performing percussion, producing a vibration that helps loosen respiratory secretions.
The other hand positions do not accomplish this task. Reduction of Risk Potential

QUESTION 280

Which is the proper hand position for performing chest vibration?

A. cup the hands
B. use the side of the hands
C. flatten the hands
D. spread the fingers of both hands

Correct Answer: C

Explanation/Reference:

The hands are flattened over the area of the body where chest percussion is used to conduct vibration through to the chest and loosen secretions. The other hand positions do not accomplish this task. Reduction of Risk Potential

QUESTION 281

Which of the following statements, if made by the parents of a newborn, does not indicate a need for further teaching about cord care?

A. "I should put alcohol on my baby's cord 34 times a day."
B. "I should put the baby's diaper on so that it covers the cord."
C. "I should call the physician if the cord becomes dark."
D. "I should wash my hands before and after I take care of the cord."

Correct Answer: D

Explanation/Reference:

Parents should be taught to wash their hands before and after providing cord care. This prevents transferring pathogens to and from the cord. Folding the diaper below the cord exposes the cord to air and allows for drying.
It also prevents wet or soiled diapers from coming into contact with the cord. Current recommendations include cleaning the area around the cord 34 times a day with a cotton swab but do not include putting alcohol or other antimicrobials on the cord. It is normal for the cord to turn dark as it dries. Health Promotion and Maintenance

QUESTION 282

The nurse is teaching parents of a newborn about feeding their infant. Which of the following instructions should the nurse include?

A. Use the defrost setting on microwave ovensto warm bottles.
B. When refrigerating formula, don't feed the baby partially used bottles after 24 hours.

C. When using formula concentrate, mix two parts water and one part concentrate.
D. If a portion of one bottle is left for the next feeding, go ahead and add new formula to fill it.

Correct Answer: A

Explanation/Reference:

Parents must be careful when warming bottles in a microwave oven because the milk can become superheated.
When a microwave oven is used, the defrost setting should be chosen, and the temperature of the formula should be checked before giving it to the baby. Refrigerated, partially used bottles should be discarded after 4 hours because the baby might have introduced some pathogens into the formula. Returning the bottle to the refrigerator does not destroy pathogens. Formula concentrate and water are usually mixed in a 1:1 ratio of one part concentrate and one part water. Infants should be offered fresh formula at each feeding. Partially used bottles should not have fresh formula added to them. Pathogens can grow in partially used bottles of formula and be transferred to the new formula. Health Promotion and Maintenance

QUESTION 283

The nurse is assessing the dental status of an 18-month-old child. How many teeth should the nurse expect to examine?

A. 6
B. 8
C. 12
D. 16

Correct Answer: C

Explanation/Reference:

In general, children begin dentition around 6 months of age. During the first 2 years of life, a quick guide to the number of teeth a child should have is as follows: Subtract the number 6 from the number of months in the age of the child. In this example, the child is 18 months old, so the formula is 18 6 = 12. An 18- month-old child should have approximately 12 teeth. Health Promotion and Maintenance

QUESTION 284

Which of the following physical findings indicates that an 1112-month-old child is at risk for developmental dysplasia of the hip?

A. refusal to walk
B. not pulling to a standing position
C. negative Trendelenburg sign
D. negative Ortolani sign

Correct Answer: B

Explanation/Reference:

The nurse might be concerned about developmental dysplasia of the hip if an 1112-month-old child doesn't pull to a standing position. An infant who does not walk by 15 months of age should be evaluated. Children should start walking between 1115 months of age. Trendelenberg sign is related to weakness of the gluteus medius muscle, not hip dysplasia. Ortolani sign is used to identify congenital subluxation or dislocation of the hip in infants. Health Promotion and Maintenance

QUESTION 285

When administering intravenous electrolyte solution, the nurse should take which of the following precautions?

A. Infuse hypertonic solutions rapidly.
B. Mix no more than 80 mEq of potassium per liter of fluid.
C. Prevent infiltration of calcium, which causes tissue necrosis and sloughing.
D. As appropriate, reevaluate the client's digitalis dosage. He might need an increased dosage because IV calcium diminishes digitalis's action.

Correct Answer: C

Explanation/Reference:

Preventing tissue infiltration is important to avoid tissue necrosis. Choice 1 is incorrect because hypertonic solutions should be infused cautiously and checked with the RN if there is a concern. Choice 2 is incorrect because potassium, mixed in the pharmacy per physician order, is mixed at a concentration no higher than 60 mEq/ L.
Physiological Adaptation